Wishing you
a long & healthy
life !

The Alternative Medicine Cabinet

*Hundreds of Ways to
Take Charge of Your Health.
Naturally.*

Kathy Gruver
MS, LMT, RM, NHC,
Doctorate in Traditional Naturopathy

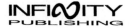

INFINITY
PUBLISHING

ii

Copyright © 2010 by Kathy Gruver

ISBN 0-7414-5903-5

Printed in the United States of America

Published March 2010

INFINITY PUBLISHING
1094 New DeHaven Street, Suite 100
West Conshohocken, PA 19428-2713
Toll-free (877) BUY BOOK
Local Phone (610) 941-9999
Fax (610) 941-9959
Info@buybooksontheweb.com
www.buybooksontheweb.com

Table of Contents

Disclaimer

This health book is not intended to prescribe or diagnose in any way. It is not meant to be a substitute for professional medical advice. Those who are sick or are experiencing any other health-related issues should consult their doctor immediately. Please note that the author is not a medical doctor and the information contained within is for educational purposes only. Please consult your physician before your begin any suggested treatment. Do not start or stop a prescription drug other than under the supervision of your doctor. Neither the author nor publisher is responsible for illness or accident caused by following the information listed here. The author assumes no responsibility if you diagnose and prescribe any treatment outlined herein without your doctor's approval.

Foreword

As a natural health professional with over two decades experience I like to share as much information with people as possible. To me, knowledge is power. As health consumers, we are overwhelmed with ads for pharmaceuticals and medical procedures but the beneficial alternative solutions are not given the same press. Over the past several years I have written numerous articles on natural health and wellness with the purpose of sharing the information I have learned.

This book is a collection of those articles along with noteworthy projects required for my master's degree. The topics range from herbs for acid reflux to hints for better sleep, from corporate health tips to how to conquer depression and anxiety naturally. I organized the articles to cover some general healing modalities first and then get into more specific needs afterwards. Since these were meant to be stand alone articles or papers, feel free to pick and choose what interests you, read them all from the beginning or randomly choose one to learn something new. Also, there will be a slight repetition of information as there are recurrent themes to healing. I hope you enjoy peering into the Alternative Medicine Cabinet.

My Perspective on Health

As an alternative health practitioner, my theory on health and wellness is that, given the right environment, the body can heal itself. The least intervention is the best bet. I also believe strongly in the mind/body connection and have seen over the years that our thoughts will manifest in our bodies. Why not hedge our bets by changing our minds, the same way we change our diets. We can have healthy bodies, but the mind and the spirit cannot be forgotten. Throughout this book, these issues are discussed.

Acknowledgments

This book is for anyone that seeks out alternatives to better their health. It is dedicated to those pioneers that were persecuted for bucking the system and challenging mainstream medicine. A salute to those rebels that risked their professional reputation, and in some cases, their lives to fight for our medical freedom and what they believed to be the truth. It's the path they forged that I can now walk down. The fight is not over, but we are gaining ground and I hope this book can be part of the solution to a growing problem.

Thanks to Kristin Anderson who made my words more clear and corrected my horrible punctuation. Also to Alyssa Boyle who put together a beautiful medicine cabinet for us to photograph.

I want to thank all my clients that hungered for knowledge and encouraged me to seek out more.

My father who always encouraged me to be the best I can be and who still to this day, believes in me.

And for my husband, Michael, who is my best friend, biggest fan and my lifelong companion. I love you.

Benefits of Massage

Massage has existed for centuries. Historians believe that hieroglyphics portraying massage were discovered in ancient Egypt in 2500 BC. A Chinese book believed to date back to the first century BCE, *The Yellow Emperor's Classic of Internal Medicine* mentions massaging the skin and flesh. What did these ancient people know? Massage feels good! But what else does it actually do? Frequently, my clients express interest in the techniques I am using and how they affect the body. Other than just plain relaxing you, here are some things that massage will do and some things that it won't do.

Research has shown massage lowers blood pressure[1] and heart rate, can lower and stabilize blood sugar[2] and moves lymph throughout your body. Okay, well, what is lymph?

Lymph is the cleansing system of the body. It runs through vessels similar to your circulatory system, but doesn't have a pump to move it (like the heart). So lymph is moved through your body by movement, breathing, muscle contraction and massage. The more the lymph moves through, the better your immune system, as the lymph carries away the "bad stuff."

When don't you want massage moving lymph? When there is cancer. The last thing you want are cancer cells being spread throughout the body. If you have cancer or have been treated for cancer, tell your massage therapist so they can make a determination if massage is right for you.

Massage helps with circulation, which is why it is so good for elderly people or those who are inactive due to

---

[1]Touch Research Institute. Originally reported in the Journal of Bodywork and Movement Therapies, January 2000, Vol. 4, No 1.

[2] www.dukemednews.com, Stress Management Can Help Control Glucose in Type 2 Diabetes, Duke University Medical Center, 2006.

injury. Massage helps move the blood and fluid around which is extraordinarily beneficial in healing. People with swollen legs and ankles like pregnant women or those with lymph edema can find relief with massage. The other benefit for the elderly is they often don't experience touch and having a weekly massage can keep their bodies and their minds healthy.

When we think of massage we think of muscles as muscles are the main part of the body that massage addresses. After a hard workout, our muscles produce toxins such as lactic acid. We want to move those out of the body to avoid muscle fatigue or pain. Massage flushes those toxins, smoothes the muscle fibers and helps relax them. Massage techniques like deep tissue and trigger point massage actually help stretch out the muscles. As a visual aid, imagine you take a rubber band and pull it taught between your hands. It's stretched out. If you have another person take one finger and push down on the middle, it stretches even more. This is essentially what massage is doing for your muscle tissue. Massage helps with muscle injuries by bringing healing blood to the area. However, avoid deep tissue massage on a muscle tear, as it can exacerbate the problem!

Massage is also used on scar tissue. When we use our muscles we get small micro tears in the tissue. That is actually how we are building bulk. When scar tissue lays down it doesn't lay flat like smooth muscle fiber. It lays cross-ways like fiberglass. Massage can help smooth out that tissue, keeping it healthy and more supple.

A technique called myofascial release can help those muscles even more by loosening up the fascia. Okay, another weird word, what is fascia? When you take the skin off a raw chicken breast, the shiny film that lies over the meat is called fascia. It lies between the muscle and skin and helps support our movements. Sometimes the fascia gets bound to muscle and restricts our range of motion. Myofascial release works on unbinding that fascia to allow us more freedom of movement.

Whereas massage used to be seen as a luxury, more and more research is demonstrating its health effects.[3] And more therapists like myself are doing medical massage. Current research shows that massage reduces nausea in cancer patients[4], decreases pain after surgery[5], reduces hospital stays in preterm infants[6], reduces anxiety and depression[7], reduces symptoms of migraine [8] and helps those suffering from fibromyalgia.[9] If you wonder if massage might be good for a condition you are faced with, contact a local massage practitioner or use your favorite search engine on the web.

We have discussed what massage does do, but what DOESN'T it do?

It does not get rid of cellulite.

Sorry, it just doesn't. It may push the fluid out of the tissue, but it will come right back. There are some "massage" techniques that use rollers and a machine to decrease it, but my understanding is that it is destined to return. Keep

[3] http://www.massagetherapy.com/learnmore/benefits.php

[4] Cassileth, Barrie, Ph.D., Vickers, Andrew, Ph.D, Memorial Sloan-Kettering Cancer Center's Integrative Medicine Service and Biostatistics Service, New York City. Originally published in Journal of Pain and Symptom Management, September 2004, Vol. 28, No. 3, pp. 244-249.

[5] JAMA and Archives Journals (2007, December 18). Massage May Help Ease Pain and Anxiety after Surgery. ScienceDaily.

[6] Journal of Perinatology (2008) 28, 815–820; doi:10.1038/jp.2008.108; published online 17 July 2008.

[7] Fields T. (2000) Touch Therapy, Churchill Livingstone. Touch Research Institute, University of Miami School of Medicine.

[8] Hernandez-Reif, M., Field, T., Dieter, J., Swerdlow. & Diego, M., (1998). Migraine headaches were reduced by massage therapy. International Journal of Neuroscience, 96, 1-11.

[9] Sunshine, W., Field, T., Schanberg, S., Quintino, O., Fierro, K., Kuhn, C., Burman, I., and Schanberg, S. (1996). Fibromyalgia benefits from massage therapy and transcutaneous electrical stimulation. Journal of Clinical Rheumatology, 2, 18-22.

drinking water and exercising which is the only thing that will help!

It doesn't give you the flu.

I have had clients say that the last time they had a massage, they got the flu. I'm not saying they didn't get the flu, I'm saying the massage didn't give it to them. What probably happened was a "healing crisis." This can happen when a lot of toxins are released at one time. Typical symptoms are headache, muscle ache, joint pain, a feeling of lethargy and all around blah. Now, as much as we don't want to feel that way, it is not a bad thing. These symptoms indicate that toxins we don't want in the body are trying to move out. To avoid the healing crisis, drink plenty of water after your massage, stretch and take a hot bath. Some people do find it beneficial to take an Ibuprofen or another anti-inflammatory. This wouldn't be my first choice, but sometimes is necessary.

Massage doesn't make you less of a man.

Seriously, I have heard men that say they don't want to have to rely on massage to make them feel good. Professional football players get massage, professional cyclists and runners get massage. Massage does not make you weak and needing or liking massage does not make you some how inferior. If it benefits you, get it. If you like it, enjoy it. Get out of your ego and get a good rub down!

As you can see, the benefits of massage clearly make it an easy option to help keep you healthier. I hope your massages are frequent and enjoyable!

Massage Sampler

As we just discussed, the benefits of massage are numerous; improved circulation, stress reduction, greater range of motion, prevention of muscle injury and it feels good. But how do you know which type of massage is right for you? Associated Bodywork & Massage Professionals (www.abmp.com), a national massage organization, estimates there are over 200 different massage techniques practiced today. I have reviewed some of the most popular massage styles and assembled them here for you. This overview is designed to help you choose the right massage for you the next time you're at your local spa or massage therapist.

Swedish, *The Basic*

Swedish, a basic technique that that is familiar to most people, is light work involving long strokes, kneading and percussion. This is usually done for relaxation and to increase circulation and is a style that is very popular amongst therapists.

Lomi Lomi, *Island Getaway*

Similar to Swedish, Lomilomi or traditional Hawaiian massage uses a lot of circular movements and forearms. Lomilomi literally means "to knead or fold."

Lymphatic Drainage, *Cleansing*

This light touch massage is used to move the lymph through the body and flush the system. This gentle technique improves metabolism, promotes the removal of toxins and encourages a healthy immune system. It is great for addressing edema or swelling and detoxification.

Hot stone, *Rock On*

In this popular spa technique the massage therapist places hot stones (up to 140 degrees Fahrenheit) on the body. The stones are then used as tools to give the massage. Pressure can be deep or light and the warmth adds to the relaxation. A note of caution: although this can feel relaxing there is increased chance of injury because inexperienced therapists cannot feel the tissue beneath their hands and can go too deep.

Deep Tissue, *Some Gusto*

Deep tissue is, just like the name implies, deeper work on the muscles. Deep tissue utilizes knuckles, elbows, feet or tools. This is another popular modality and is useful for aches, knots, tension and muscle pain. Contrary to popular belief, this doesn't have to hurt. If the pressure is too much during your massage, ask your therapist to lighten up. A good therapist will listen and should never try to convince you that they know better.

Sports massage, *Game On*

Sports massage is a combination of techniques specifically for the athlete. Very useful for pre and post event, sports massage stretches, kneads, shakes and uses deep pressure to help prevent and address injuries. Post event massage can calm the nervous system and helps to flush the lactic acid out of the muscles, reducing recovery time.

Trigger Point, *Get to the Root of the Problem*

Trigger points are portions of the muscle fibers that have gone into spasm. Similar to deep tissue massage, the therapist searches out specific trigger points which refer pain to other parts of the body. This technique is based on two decades of research and was made popular in the 1980s by doctors who mapped the trigger points and their referral patterns. Therapists use this technique for pain management, increased range of motion and rehabilitation after injuries. A great resource is *Myofascial Pain and Dysfunction; A Trigger Point Manual* by Travell and Simons, 1983.

Shiatsu, *A Taste of Japan*

Shiatsu works with energy meridians similar to those used in Acupuncture. It is performed on the floor and the client stay fully clothed. Shiatsu isn't just about the physical. It is used to tone and balance the energy and to calm or activate the body's systems. This technique is very versatile. The compression used during shiatsu can be deeper in a pre-sport situation or lighter to help drain lymph. Instead of focusing on specific muscle groups, Shiatsu focuses on the intention and the energy.

Acupressure is similar to shiatsu with the exception that it focuses on individual points, not whole energy meridians and can be used for self-treatment.

Thai, *Lazy Man's Yoga*

Thai massage, popular in modern spas, has been taught and practiced in Thailand for 2,500 years. This technique is performed on the floor, fully clothed and utilizes a lot of stretching and manipulating of the client's limbs and torso. This can be physically intense so it is not recommended for people with injuries. This technique is traditionally done on the floor, but many spas are offering a variety called table Thai. Specify which you are getting if you are looking for this type of massage. You might be surprised.

Barefoot, *Step on the Wild Side*

Barefoot or Compressive Deep Tissue is a massage practice that uses the therapist's feet instead of hands. Although similar techniques have been used in other countries for centuries, this American style grew out of a need for deeper, continuous pressure with less stress on the therapist's hands and arms. This approach is performed on the floor with the client clothed. The only downside to this technique is you cannot get as much detail work with the feet as you can with the hands and there is increased chance of injury with an inexperienced therapist.

Reflexology, *More Than a Foot Massage*

Reflexology, typically done on the feet but also popular on the hands and ears, follows a belief that every point on the body has a corresponding point on the foot. An ancient Chinese therapy, reflexology is especially useful for stress-related illness and emotional disorders. However, over time this diagnostic and therapeutic system has become less clinical and more relaxing.

Medical Massage, *The New Kid*

This is a category of massage, not really a technique on its own and is relatively new. It is used for injuries or rehabilitation and indicates that the therapist has training to address specific pathologies such as frozen shoulder, carpal tunnel, sciatica, disease states and others. These therapists often work with Chiropractors, Physical Therapists and Doctors. Some therapists use "medical massage" as a general term that differentiates their technique from "spa massage."

Reiki, *Spirit Calling*

Reiki is a technique that a lot of massage therapists utilize but it is not really a type of massage. Reiki (meaning Universal Life Force) is a hands-on healing technique that uses universal energy flowing through a practitioner into the person being healed. It heals on all levels of body, mind and spirit and is a great addition to a massage or as a stand alone session. (See page 18 for a full description)

Rolfing, *Intention*

Rich Goodstein, an advanced Rolfer for 28 years explains that Rolfing is not really a massage technique.

"Rolfing works globally, with range of motion, breath and realigning the body. It's useful to help the body surrender and let go of patterns." Contrary to popular misconception, Rolfing doesn't have to be deep and does not have to hurt. "Sure," Rich goes on to say, "it can make you sore just like yoga class or Pilates can." Unlike massage, Rolfing is done in sessions of 10 or sometimes 15 and works on unifying the whole body, including the emotions.

I hope this brief exploration of massage techniques proves helpful. Whichever massage you choose, may they be frequent and beneficial.

Communication with Your Massage Therapist

Communication is defined as *the science or practice of transmitting information.*[10] But just as important as transmitting information is receiving and processing it. When working with people such as a massage therapist or natural health professional, clear communication, both verbal and non-verbal is key to getting the experience you are seeking.

Communication doesn't start when you get on the table. Before you even meet the therapist you have an opportunity to implement clear communication skills.

~ Check on price and the amount of time you get for that price. It might be advantageous to see if you have the option of going longer at the time of the massage.

~ Find out the cancellation and no-show policy and adhere to it if you must cancel.

~ Tell the therapist why you are coming to see them and the results that you expect. This can save you disappointment, time and money, as they might not even specialize in what you are looking for.

~ Once the appointment has been made, make sure you have their address and correct directions/parking instructions. Ask for their cell phone number and get specific instructions to their office if you need them. And please be respectful and write it down, don't assume you will remember. If they are coming to you, give them your address and any unusual parking information like street cleaning on certain days, etc.

---

[10] The Oxford Essential Dictionary. 1998 Oxford University Press, pg. 114.

Once you meet the therapist, clear communication of your expectations and needs is crucial.

~ Most therapists want to know how you found them and appreciate it if you volunteer that information.

~ Fill out the intake form completely and bring to their attention anything particularly unusual or that needs explanation.

~ Mention any illnesses, injuries, previous surgeries, bumps, bruises, cuts or herpes outbreaks. (This last item might be embarrassing, but is important nonetheless as the therapist is vulnerable to contracting it by touching any sores.)

~ Tell them how you like your pressure, if there is anything that needs to be avoided or if you would like them to focus on a particular area or issue.

If you are a first-timer, you'll want to find out how this therapist works. For example, do you disrobe completely or do they prefer underwear to be left on. It's okay to be nervous your first time and to even share this feeling with the therapist. Your therapist can typically sense your discomfort, and will do their best to make you feel relaxed and comfortable.

~ If you're not familiar with massage have them explain some of the benefits and tell them specifically what you expect. For example, "I have really bad headaches, I'm looking for some relief." Or "I really just want to relax and unwind."

If the therapist asks you, "How are you feeling?" Be as specific as possible with your answers so the therapist can address what ails you. Answers like "Fine." or "I feel bad." do little to enlighten the therapist to your specific needs.

~ If you have had massage before, it's perfectly acceptable to tell the new therapist what you liked and didn't like about the last therapist. I have had therapists shove their oily fingers in my ears. I don't like that. Who would? I tell every new therapist NOT to do that to me.

~ And if you like to have your massage in silence, saying that up front is a good idea. Don't assume the therapist will pick up on it once the massage has started.

~ Make it clear if you need to have anything adjusted once the massage has begun such as the temperature, the music, and the pressure. They should change whatever is not working for you. It's your time and the treatment should be personalized for you.

~ Many spas automatically use hot towels. If this is something you prefer to not have, ask if this is part of their treatment and tell the therapist you would like to skip it.

~ Tell the therapist if you'd like a whole body massage or if you just want certain areas concentrated upon. Sometimes if you mention certain tension spots, the practitioner may get carried away and run out of time for the rest of your body. You might be okay with that or want work elsewhere. Clarify so they know.

After the massage:

~ Ask questions if you have them.

~ It is important to drink water and do light stretching.

~ Reschedule another appointment. Some therapists like myself get very booked and you may have to wait several weeks for an appointment if you don't rebook immediately.

~ Remember that permanent changes rarely occur with the first session, so you may need more work.

~ If you have had deep work, you may be sore and ice might be appropriate.

~ If you want to become a regular client, ask if you can have a standing appointment or if there is a price break for buying more than one. Many therapists will give you discounts for purchasing a series, such as 10% off or buy five get the sixth free.

In order to receive the most benefit from massage, you need to feel comfortable and relaxed. A big part of this is developing a sense of trust and understanding between you and your therapist. In such a personal relationship as massage, we can see how interpersonal communication can make or break this experience. Be open and concise, truly listen, choose your words carefully and remember more information is better than none.

14

Homeopathy

Let's move from talk of the body,
to the subtle energies of the body.

With so many Americans turning to alternative medicine in the past several years, we are hearing more about homeopathics. But what is Homeopathy? Hopefully this will clear up the mystique.

The American Heritage Science Dictionary defines homeopathy *as a nontraditional system for treating and preventing disease, in which minute amounts of a substance that in large amounts causes disease symptoms are given to healthy individuals. This is thought to enhance the body's natural defenses.*

Classical Homeopathy involves comprehensive questioning and analysis of a patient's symptoms (through an in-depth interview and questionnaire) and the physical, emotional and spiritual responses to each disorder. For example, a headache would be examined in regards to what brought it on, what makes it better or worse, if there is a time of day that aggravates it, is it limited to a certain part of the head, what were the circumstances that caused it, etc. Classical homeopathy is most often used to treat a specific disease or symptom. In this type of practice, one remedy at a time is given. Some practitioners are of the belief that the combination remedies commonly found in drug stores are less effective, if effective at all.

Constitutional Homeopathy treats the root personality of each patient. It can be described as a remedy which covers the totality of a patient's mental and physical characteristics over a long period of time, excluding temporary changes during an acute illness. Constitutional homeopathy, in contrast to classical, is not necessarily used to treat a specific symptom, but to balance the whole being and promote homeostasis. There is a belief that we cannot actually change our constitution, but that we can develop a healthier, more positive version of it.

How to find the Correct Remedy: Regardless of what type of homeopathy you are utilizing, the correct remedy is determined by an in-depth interview or a questionnaire. The prescribing therapist may ask you more probing questions about the symptoms, your childhood, your parents, etc. It is not always easy to find the correct remedy, but when it is selected, a change can be seen almost immediately. Didier Grandgeorge in his book, *The Spirit of Homeopathic Medicine* states, "For each homeopathic remedy we have tried to find the dominant idea representing the problem that the individual is confronting at the unconscious level. By studying in this way the whole range of physical and mental symptoms of an ill person, we discover the homeopathic remedy that covers the totality of symptoms." [11]

The homeopathic practitioner must not only choose the right remedy, but prescribe the appropriate dosage. If you are self-prescribing and buying homeopathic medicine in the store, you will either get a combination remedy or a very low dose (30X or 30C). By law in the United States, the higher potencies are only available through homeopathic practitioners. Some diseases react better to different potencies and it is therefore important to discuss what the dosage will be, how often you should repeat it and what to do if the symptoms return or new symptoms appear.

Most homeopaths believe that certain substances will counteract the effect of the medications. For example, coffee, camphor, toothpaste and marijuana should not be used while you are taking homeopathics. They also recommend waiting 15 minutes before and after taking a dosage before eating or drinking anything. Also, most practitioners will encourage

---

[11] Grandgeorge, Didier. (1998). The Spirit of Homeopathic Medicine. North Atlantic Books, Berkeley.

patients to stop any prescription medications if possible. This can cause problems, as most allopathic (traditional Western) physicians don't understand or acknowledge the value of homeopathics. Try to be open with your doctor though and don't ever stop prescription medication without alerting them first.

Homeopathic medications come in several forms: liquid, sugar pills and lactose pills. Never handle the medicine directly. Either drip the liquids into water or your mouth (don't touch the dropper with your lips), and with the pills, empty the correct amount into the cap and then put straight into your mouth.

The Holistic Approach to Homeopathy. Homeopathy is not a "one size fits all" system of medicine like we experience with our prescription-happy Western practitioners. Through the use of the above mentioned interview and questionnaire, the practitioner can find the remedy that is right for you. Two people could come into the office; both feeling depressed and walk out with two very different, perhaps opposite remedies. If the first remedy you are given doesn't work, another remedy is available for you to try. The communicative nature of the homeopathic practice builds a relationship of trust between patient and doctor. Through using Homeopathics, physical dis-ease can be treated as well as emotional and spiritual issues. Symptoms are not just covered up as often happens in Western medicine.

The Benefits of Choosing a Homeopathic Approach. The benefits of homeopathy are numerous. One benefit is that there are no adverse side effects as there can be with prescription medication, thus it is totally appropriate for children (see pg. 48 for more information on homeopathics and children), pregnant women and even pets. The patient may have a temporary worsening of symptoms while the body adjusts to the remedy but this is usually fleeting. In some cases, the patient may even experience old symptoms in reverse order as the homeopathic remedies work to clear the whole body. For example, the asthma may clear, but the sinus problems from years ago may return then go away. Then another ailment from the past will return, and go away. This pattern may repeat until all ailments are resolved and true healing occurs. This is a positive sign, as symptoms disappear in the order they showed up. They should also move from inside out, so the stomach ache may resolve, but old skin problems might show up temporarily.

Another benefit is that homeopathy is individualized medicine exclusive to each patient which is in direct contrast to Western medicine.

Other benefits are that the remedies are quite affordable and abundant. According to Grandgeorge, "One single gram of mother tincture of Arnica provides enough Arnica 15 CH to treat the entire human race." [12]

Another advantage is that homeopathy can produce lasting change in the body. It is not a temporary cessation of symptoms; it helps the body truly heal itself.

Store Bought vs. Practitioner Formulated Remedies. Although combination remedies are readily available in health food stores it is recommended that you see a qualified practitioner when integrating homeopathics in order to get the specific remedy to address your exact needs.

The drawback of combination remedies labeled with symptoms such as "headache" or "PMS" is that they are formulated with the most common remedies to treat that particular ailment, when only one or two might really be needed for your particular set of symptoms.

Though Homeopathy might seem fringe to you, there are many studies and successes to back it up. Why not give it a chance? It's affordable and there aren't any side effects, so you have nothing to lose. Its effectiveness might just surprise you!

---

[12] Grandgeorge, Didier. (1998). The Spirit of Homeopathic Medicine. North Atlantic Books, Berkeley.

Reiki: A Modern Oral Tradition

Reiki is a hands-on healing energy technique where universal energy or chi comes through the practitioner and into the person being healed. It heals on all levels of body, mind and spirit. It is relaxing, balancing and strengthening.

I had my first Reiki attunement in 1994 from a teacher in Los Angeles. An attunement is another name for the initiation/procedure to give the healer the ability to use Reiki. An attunement consists of symbols placed in the hands and head of the soon-to-be healer. The attunement itself is a quick process, taking only a few minutes, but most Reiki teachers spend several hours if not days with the practitioner before the actual attunement.

There are three levels of Reiki: I, II and III (master level). The first level gives you the ability to practice on yourself and others. The second provides you with symbols to enhance the practice and also work from a distance, and the third attunement teaches you how to teach others. That is called the master level and unlike the name implies, does not make someone at that level superior to others at the lower stages. It simply means that they can pass attunements and teach others.

Reiki, meaning Universal Light Energy, is thought to be as ancient as mankind itself and its roots are steeped in myth. It is based on a master/teacher relationship and on the initiation of the students. Reiki was re-discovered by a man that was looking for answers. Mikao Usui, a Christian minister and university professor, wanted to know how Jesus did his healing. A ten year quest abroad and a seven year search in the United States proved useless. Usui decided to embark on another journey.

He returned to Japan where he studied ancient texts in a Zen Monastery but knew he needed to go through the "test." The test was a three week fast and meditation. On the final morning of his quest, slightly before sunrise, Usui saw a bolt of light coming from the sky directly towards him. He felt fear and wanted to run but realized that is what he had been waiting for. The light struck his forehead over his third eye and Usui lost consciousness. He saw millions of colorful bubbles and the Reiki symbols appeared to him along with information about how to use them. It was the first Reiki attunement.

Usui took Reiki through the streets of Japan and spent the next several years traveling, healing, and sharing his story. It was believed that Usui made 16-18 Reiki masters in his career but only Dr. Hayashi was mentioned in most Reiki sources and was considered Usui's successor. Dr. Hayashi went on to teach Reiki, open a healing clinic and made sixteen masters in his lifetime.

Although once kept secret, information on Reiki is now readily available in every book store and on countless websites including EBay. What remains unique about Reiki is that you must have someone teach you. You can read all the books you want, but without the hands-on attunement, it just won't work. I do believe that some people are born with Reiki ability, but I still think having a teacher as a guide is necessary. It helps you to hone your skill and provides you with more focus and intention.

How Reiki works is pretty simple. You place your hands on the person (or a few inches above the body) with the intention of healing, and the energy starts to flow. It usually feels like a heat and tingling in the hands. There is often a deep sense of relaxation for the person enjoying the session and they may even fall asleep. Sometimes laughter or tears come too. Reiki can only be used for positive purposes and cannot you harm in any way. It enhances and accelerates the body's healing ability and balances the chi.

Most people who practice Reiki are in the healing arts, but many lay people learn it to help with family, friends or personal development. Reiki is great for children, plants and animals. It can help with emotional healing after a loss or breakup, physical healing to speed the process and on a spiritual level to provide grounding or focus. Reiki practitioners exist in practically every city in the world and are easy to locate on the internet or in health-related publications.

If you are looking for a Reiki healing session, ask the practitioner how long they have been practicing and what level they have been taught. Some use crystals and other accoutrements like certain pieces of jewelry or clothing. Ask what their healing involves in advance and if you're not comfortable with their technique, look elsewhere. People used to put great importance on if they could trace their lineage to one of the original teachers. Though it is not as important these days, you should know what the healer's background is and where they studied. Make sure you connect with them and trust them, or seek another healer.

If you want to learn Reiki, seek out a seasoned, level three master. Someone should not be teaching others without years of practice. Ask if your attunement involves a healing session first and if handouts are included. Also, make sure they can give you a certificate, especially if you want to be a practitioner yourself. You may want to meet the person before committing to the attunement, and if you don't feel a good connection, seek guidance elsewhere. There are now many versions of Reiki with slightly different symbols, different names, and different methods. A more regimented group believes Reiki should be exclusive and expensive. Others give hundreds of people attunements in a weekend at a campsite. For $75 you can become a Reiki Master on EBay, though this approach is not recommended as it contradicts the person to person attunement principles previously mentioned. Reiki is becoming more mainstream and even hospitals and cancer centers are now embracing Reiki's healing and research is being carried out on its success rates.

I wish you all luck on your search for healing.

Nutrition: Kathy's Top 10 Picks

This was a project required for my master's degree and was based on the information found in one specific book, *The 150 Healthiest Foods on Earth* by Jonny Bowden, PhD, CNS. The page numbers used are in the footnotes. What follows is my top 10 healthy foods list with many more that could have been added.

Blueberries

Blueberries topped my list as one of the most potent antioxidants and anti-inflammatories you can consume which helps combat the oxidative stress that can cause Alzheimer's, Parkinson's, diabetes, heart disease, and arthritis associated with inflammation. They are high in polyphenols which turn on neurons in the brain, improve motor coordination, reduce eye strain, improve night vision and prevent macular degeneration. Blueberries are the ultimate memory food.[13]

Blueberries were tested to have one of the highest ORAC (Oxygen Radical Absorbance Capacity) values of all times which means they are very high in the above mentioned antioxidants. These tasty berries also contain pterostilbene which helps in regulating fatty acid metabolism and fats in the blood stream. They have also been shown to be cancer preventing. This is such an easy food to add to your diet; having a handful as a snack or putting them on cereals or yogurt. I believe locally grown organic fruit is best and should be chosen whenever possible. This is the representative fruit on my list and will complement the other foods providing vitamins, antioxidants and phytochemicals.

---

[13] Page 101

Wild Caught Salmon

Wild caught salmon is my next choice, which is also popular among the experts. Salmon is high in omega 3 fatty acids which benefit heart and brain health as well as inflammation, circulation, memory, thought and blood sugar control.[14] It is a high quality protein, containing potassium and cancer-fighting selenium as well as the vitamins B12 and niacin. I have friends that have sworn off fish because of the high mercury content. This is certainly something to be concerned about but for the most part, the health benefits far outweigh the mercury risk. Also, selenium which is contained in salmon is a powerful chelator of mercury[15] and salmon is one of the least mercury toxic fish. However, it is recommended that pregnant women avoid fish for the first six months of pregnancy while the fetus is in its most sensitive phases of development.

However, and this is a BIG however, you should only eat wild caught salmon. Farm raised salmon is bad for many reasons. It has fewer omega 3s and more omega 6s of which we don't need as much. They are also high in dangerous PCBs (Polychlorinated Biphenyls). Wild salmon gets its wonderful pink color from the krill it naturally consumes. Farmed salmon, which is grain fed, is dyed pink (chosen by using a color wheel like at a paint store) and who knows what long term effect that will have on us. Also, the fish at farms are packed in very close to each other, creating a breeding ground for disease.

Broccoli

One of my two vegetable suggestions is broccoli. Not only is broccoli one of the least contaminated foods with pesticides[16] but it is filled with massive amounts of potassium, protein, fiber, calcium, vitamins C and A, folate,

---

[14] Page 216

[15] Page 219

[16] Page 25

magnesium, phosphorus, and beta-carotene. Plus, it contains lutein and zeaxanthin, which have been shown to reduce and prevent macular degeneration. Broccoli also has some cancer-preventing strength. It is high in a phytochemical called isothiocyanates, which neutralize carcinogens. They help prevent lung and esophageal cancers and may lower the risk of other cancers like gastrointestinal.

Indole-3-carbinol, a strong antioxidant and stimulator of beneficial enzymes helps protect DNA and reduces the risk of breast and cervical cancer by increasing the ratio of "good" estrogen metabolites to "bad." It also protects against the carcinogenic effects of pesticides and other toxins. Broccoli is easy to prepare and is the perfect addition to any meal. Avoid the heavy cheese sauce though and enjoy the pure green goodness of broccoli.

Garlic

Garlic is one of the oldest medicinal foods on the planet.[17] It is lipid lowering, anti-thrombotic, anti-blood coagulation, and antihypertensive, an antioxidant, antimicrobial, antiviral, anti-parasitic, and tasty. It lowers overall cholesterol, raises HDL (the good stuff), reduces plaque, decreases risk of stomach and colon cancer, inhibits leukemia, and wards off colds (and vampires). It helps regulate blood pressure and is believed to help with weight control. There have been numerous studies on garlic and it has been shown that it must be crushed or chopped to release its full potential.[18] Allicin is the healthy compound that is responsible for most of the health benefits that are released when "damaged." Eating garlic raw isn't recommended because it can be hard on the stomach and most supplements just don't do this little guy justice. Add garlic to your salmon, broccoli, spinach and just about anything else on my

[17] Page 282
[18] Page 283

list, except perhaps the blueberries! Avoid microwaving, as it destroys its goodness all together.

Olive Oil

It is so easy to add beneficial olive oil to your diet. It can be added to almost anything and is a great cooking medium. It is high in omega 3 fats, and phenols which are antioxidants, and oleic acid, which is a heart-healthy monounsaturated fat. Olive oil has been shown to lower LDL (the bad stuff), raise HDL (the good stuff) and decrease the need for blood pressure medications by 48%. Four tablespoons a day are recommended and have been shown to decrease the risk of colon and bowel cancer.

Olive is one of the few oils that can be consumed in its crude form with no processing[19] so it is recommended that you get extra virgin oil only, which is the first press of the olives. Not refining the oil keeps the benefits of conserving the vitamins, essential fatty acids, antioxidants and other nutrients. Olive oil is also good on your skin and many people use it after their shower to help moisturize and pamper the skin. Since olive oil is so easy to cook with, it mixes well with my other food choices.

Eggs

Eggs are considered by Bowden as nature's most perfect food.[20] It is a great source of protein and contains all nine essential amino acids. Eggs are a wonderful source of vitamins and minerals and are the best source for choline which assists with cardiovascular and brain function, cell membrane health and prevents the accumulation of fat and cholesterol in the liver. It also forms a compound which lowers homecysteine, a risk factor for heart disease and helps with liver detoxification. It's thought to protect against

---

[19] Page 303
[20] Page 191

diseases associated with aging like dementia and Alzheimer's disease.

Eggs are also high in lutein and zeoxanthin which are important for eye health. Eating eggs and spinach together is a great way to help absorb of that lutein which needs fat for absorption. In a recent study, eggs have been shown to help prevent breast cancer.[21] And women who ate six eggs a week as opposed to two showed a lowered risk of breast cancer by 44 percent. Eggs also contain trace amounts of more than fifteen vitamins and minerals including cancer-fighting selenium and a high sulfur content that helps promotes healthy hair and nails.

It is recommended to eat eggs poached, boiled or raw. Breaking and cooking the yolk oxidizes it and can lead to health issues especially from eggs that have been sitting out for a long time (avoid that breakfast buffet). For those that are concerned about salmonella from raw eggs, experts say that only about .03% of all eggs are contaminated and if you eat cage free eggs the incidence drops even more. Recently eggs have been enriched with Omega 3 fatty acids which are a boon to health. Dr. Bowden also mentions the health obsession with egg whites. He sites a study done by Harvard that it's <u>never</u> been shown that people who eat more eggs have more heart attacks than anyone else.[22]

Spinach

Spinach and eggs could be the perfect breakfast meal. Spinach provides more nutrients than almost any food on the planet. Spinach is high in vitamin K, calcium, magnesium, vitamin D, manganese, folic acid, iron, C, and quercitin. Vitamin D is very important and helps to build strong bones and anchors calcium in the body. I recently listened to a lecture on vitamin D that mentioned it's one of the most

---

[21] Page 192

[22] Page 193

deficient vitamins in the United States; we can get more with some spinach!

Spinach is high in flavonoids which function as antioxidant and anticancer agents. Flavonoids reduce skin cancers, reduce division in stomach cancer cells, lessen the incidence of breast cancer, fight prostate cancer, and cause cancer cells to self-destruct. Vitamins C and A prevent cholesterol from becoming oxidized, sticking together and building up in arteries. They reduce inflammation and protect the brain against age-related disorders like dementia. Folic acid decreases homocysteine, which is harmful to blood vessels and increases the risk for stroke and heart disease. Spinach lowers blood pressure and protects the heart with magnesium. Spinach is also high in iron which is good for all of us, especially menstruating women. Finally, spinach contains lutein, which helps protect eyes from cataracts and macular degeneration. It is one of the lowest calorie foods around.[23] Conventionally grown spinach was listed as high in pesticides, so buy organic and wash well.

Avocado

Avocado is one of my favorite foods even though I had never even seen one until I moved to California. It is a perfect snack that comes in its own little cup and is high in monounsaturated fat and oleic acid (an omega 9) which lowers cholesterol. Studies involving avocados showed that participant's LDL went down and HDL went up and they saw a drop in total cholesterol. Avocados are also high in beta-sitosterol which lowers cholesterol and protects the prostate gland. The monounsaturated fat in avocados has been linked to a reduced risk of cancer and diabetes. Avocados are a good source of fiber, containing between 11 and 17 grams, plus potassium, folate, vitamin A, beta-carotene and beta-cryptoxanthin, and lutein, which is good

---

[23] Page 61

for eye health and glowing skin.[24] California avocados have fewer calories than the Florida variety and less fat and carbohydrates, but Florida's contain more potassium. Adding avocados to eggs and salads is a great way to get the benefits from this fruit.

Filtered Water

We cannot survive without clean healthy drinking water. And boy has it been making the news lately; water contaminated with pharmaceuticals, bottled water turning out to be just tap water, water on airplanes contaminated with feces. It's obviously a hot button topic and absolutely made my top 10 list.

Our bodies are 83% water and it's necessary for every single metabolic action in the body. It flushes fat and toxins out, helps us digest and absorb nutrients and vitamins, improves energy, increases mental and physical performance, keeps our skin healthy and glowing, and can help you lose weight. It lubricates and cushions joints, and if dehydrated, you are more susceptible to ailments. Water reduces cramping of the muscles and early onset of fatigue. Studies show that people with high intake of water have significantly lower risk for fatal coronary heart disease.[25]

No one knows for sure where the eight glasses a day rule came from, but Dr. Bowden suggests taking your weight, dividing it in half and drinking that number of ounces a day. [26] It is extremely important to know the source of your drinking water. It is recommended in the book to NEVER drink tap water. And this is where politics comes into play. Since the government determines what is safe and they are pressured by companies that are dumping/leaking unsafe things, where does the truth lie? I am personally skeptical of food and water regulations established by the

---

[24] Page 97

[25] Page 269

[26] Page 271

government, and I make sure that to seek out reputable bottled water. It just seems a safer choice.

<u>Red Wine</u>

With a husband who is a food and wine writer, red wine had to make my list. It is high in the antioxidant resveratrol, which is beneficial in preventing harmful elements in the body from attacking healthy cells and is also a great anti-aging compound.[27] Red wine can prevent heart disease and help reduce lung tissue inflammation such as in COPD (Chronic Obstructive Pulmonary Disease). Red wine can raise HDL cholesterol and lower risk of heart attack, and may prevent more if you've already had one. It may also help prevent blood clots and reduce blood vessel damage caused by fat deposits.

Although consumption of red wine in moderation clearly has health benefits, there are conflicting studies on its effects on breast cancer. One study shows benefits, the other shows an increase in incidence. I would like to see more studies and in the mean time I'm not giving up my Merlot. If it is proven that breast cancer rates increase with consumption of alcohol, studies show that consuming folic acid can make the problem with breast cancer and alcohol consumption lessen.[28]

The health benefits of red wine are not license to over consume, for some segments of our population, even one sip is not a good idea. Let's face it; some people should not be drinking. Alcoholism is one of the biggest problems in our society and even a sip of wine can put some people over the edge.

Moderation is the key to receiving the health benefits of red wine. Too much alcohol can raise triglycerides, increase blood pressure and lead to weight gain, not to mention the possibility of drunk driving, spousal abuse and

---

[27] Page 262

[28] Page 263

missed work days. But if drinking is something that a person can do intelligently, then pop the cork and enjoy the healthy benefits of the nectar of the gods. Dr. Bowden states that no pregnant woman should drink, [29] with which I slightly disagree. I think a small amount of wine or champagne is fine in the final trimester.

The only other thing I would add to my list is to eat these foods in their most natural state. No matter how healthy they are, if they are charred to death and then covered in a heavy sauce, the benefits decrease. Choose organic, locally grown products whenever possible. Select whole foods over processed ones and remember with every swipe of a product code in a grocery store, we cast our vote. Eat, Drink and Be Healthy!

All References came from *The 150 Healthiest Foods on Earth*, Dr. Jonny Bowden, PhD, CNS, 2007, Fair Winds Press.

---

[29] Page 263

An Herbal Overview

Herbs are a valuable source of natural medicine. Vitamins and minerals from herbs have been used safely for centuries. Many prescription drugs have their origins in herbal medicine. Aspirin for example, is derived from white willow bark. The advantage of herbal medicine is you get the whole compound, which often eliminates any side effects that might be present if it is broken down and turned into a prescription or over the counter drug.

There is certainly some overlap amongst herbal traditions but there is a large distinction between Chinese and American herbal therapy. Ayurveda (Traditional Indian Medicine) also utilizes an herbal system of medicine. There are many premade individual and combination herbal formulas so you don't have to feel responsible for concocting your own. It is important to remember that these are chemical compounds and may interact with other drugs or may need to be eliminated before surgery. Make sure you inform your medical team of any herbs that you are taking. You can also reference the book *A-Z Guide to Drug-Herb-Vitamin Interactions* (copyright 2006 by Healthnotes, Inc). Like other natural health remedies, herbs encourage the body to heal itself and activate the natural powers that we possess. Here are some common ways to take herbs.

- Capsule: Gelatin capsule containing powdered or chopped herbs that are typically unpleasant to take directly by mouth. Most commercially available herbs are given this way.

- Compress: A pad or cotton dipped in herbs that have been boiled in water. Good for swelling, pain, etc.

- Infusion: Pouring hot liquid over the herb, steeping and drinking as a tea.

- Poultice: Warm mashed or ground herbs applied directly to the skin.

- Tincture: Another common way to find commercially prepared herbs, this involves soaking the herbs in an alcohol base, straining them, then taking the extracted liquid by mouth or using externally. This is a convenient way to take the herbs and they have a long shelf life with this preparation as the alcohol preserves the herbs. You can also buy herbs in bulk and make your own tinctures at home.

To make your own tinctures take an ounce of whole or cut herbs and put in a glass container with lid. I recommend glass instead of plastic since plastic can leech into the tincture. Cover the herbs with alcohol - I typically use vodka. Put the lid on and shake twice daily for two weeks. Strain the mixture and bottle the liquid.

The method you use to take herbs is entirely up to you and what is available in your area. Most cities now have an herbal shop where you can buy herbs in bulk and take them any way you'd like. Some do have a less than desirable taste and may be better in capsules or tinctures. Many garden stores have potted herbs that you can grow at home and you can probably find seeds to most common herbs on line. If you want to make your own teas, empty tea bags are available that you stuff and seal with an iron. You could also use a tea ball commonly found in kitchen stores.

If you'd like to make your own capsules, this is easy to do as well. I recommend getting the herbs in powdered form or using a coffee grinder to make the particles smaller. You can either put the ingredients in a bowl and just fill and close the empty capsules, or you can get a capsule maker, which is affordable and readily available on line. They typically hold 25 or 50 capsule halves. You pour the herbs across the tops until the half capsules fill. Then, place the other half on top to seal the capsule. It sounds complicated, but it's easier to use this when making a lot of doses.

There are some good herbal books available and on-line resources abound. Remember to double check your sources, make sure the herbs won't interfere with any prescriptions and know that herbs are chemicals and will react in the body so don't assume they are safe just because they are natural.

As a side note: Many people self-prescribe when it comes to herbs. Where in most cases that is safe, I recommend doing in-depth research, talking to a professional herbalist or health practitioner or taking herb classes.

Bach Flower Essences

In the 1930's Edward Bach, a medical doctor and bacteriologist, developed a healing system, which he named Bach Flower Essences. He used 38 individual flowers plus a combination of five flowers he called *Rescue Remedy*. Dr. Bach's healing theories were cutting edge for the time, and are studied and widely used today by naturopathic practitioners and individuals. He believed that every person had the ability to heal themselves and that anyone could use the flower remedies. He chose plants with, what he believed had a high vibration, and expected them to heal through that vibration. He ignored physical symptoms, instead focusing on disharmonies of energy. To him, the principles of unity, perfection and harmony meant more than disease, dysfunction and sickness. Dr. Bach's healing strategy was "Don't fight it, transform it" and he achieved this through his simple remedies.

The essences work on the emotional state of the person, transforming the negative into positive. These negative states, if not addressed, can manifest as disease in the body. Although Bach Flower Essences do not directly address physical issues, they can stave off illness through balancing the spiritual/emotional state. They are homeopathically prepared, which means there are no chemical aspects of the plant left. They work strictly on an energetic level.

To use the remedies, a questionnaire is filled out by the client and the chosen remedies are determined by those answers. I equate this to the keys on the piano. We are all born with emotional "notes." Life experiences pound on certain keys such as an alcoholic father, abusive step-parent, mental illness in the family, early losses, etcetera. These events bang on the keys and overtime, they get out of tune. Flower essences come in and retune our emotional piano.

The chosen essences are mixed into a master bottle, which are to be taken four times per day. It is not recommended to use more than seven flowers at a time. Often the emotions unfold like an onion and as you balance some emotional states different ones will appear. It's good to reevaluate the formula after a few weeks and change what is necessary to address evolving emotional issues. I have noticed that people will suddenly stop taking the remedy or lose it. That seems to be an indication that a new formula is needed.

There are numerous advantages to Bach Flower Essences:

- You get quick results. I've seen change in a matter of hours. Rescue Remedy works very quickly and has gotten me through two weddings, one divorce, numerous funerals, near car accidents, and a knife wound in my hand.

- They are affordable. Each remedy costs about $14 and can be found at health food stores and online. You can also purchase the full series of remedies to mix for yourself and others. That runs between $415 and $465 depending on whether you want the stylish leather case.

- If it doesn't work for you, there are no side effects. It simply won't do anything.

- The essences don't interact with other medications or therapies, though you should still tell your physician you are taking them.

- You can do it yourself, though the input and expertise of a trained professional is always recommended.

- They are great for kids and pets. I had a client that used rescue remedy for her nervous horse; she would just put it in his water. They now make alcohol free Rescue Remedy for pets and kids. If alcohol is a problem for you, place in warm water to evaporate the alcohol.

- Bach Flower Essences are customized medicine, not one-size-fits-all therapy. There are millions of combinations that could be made from those 38 flowers. For example there are at least five different remedies that can be chosen for depression depending on the cause and type.

When I recommend flower essences for clients I have them fill out the questionnaire. I review their answers, ask more questions and try to determine what the best combination will be for them. I mix the formula and give them a hand out that tells them what flowers are in the formula, what conditions they are being used for, directions on how to take it and I also include empowering statements or affirmations. I often recommend certain activities like gardening, deep breathing, walking or vigorous exercise depending on the symptoms and the formula. (See example form below.)

The consultation can be done over the phone, but in person is better to observe body language and physical reaction during the interview. I follow up with the client in a few days and we reevaluate in two weeks. Usually I change the formula at that time.

Excerpt from real protocol.

Centaury: Neglecting your own needs and difficulty saying no (what the flower is for)

Anytime anyone asks for something ask "What are their real motives?" "What do I really want?" (The first phrases are recommendations, the next are affirmations)

"I am solely responsible for my own development"
"I stand up for my own needs"

Elm: Overwhelmed

Provide more breaks when planning your work
"I am up to the situation"
"I always have the help I need"

Oak: Sense of duty, neglect own needs
*   Do exercises for neck and shoulder area*
*   "I shall do it"*
*   "Energy is flowing to me from the primal source"*

Dr. Bach's essences are not the only ones out there; there are other similar protocols to be found. Australian Bush Flowers are another popular group that uses between 65 and 69 essences from Australian flowers. I have found others that were invented and mixed by individuals. Practitioners can range from the self-taught to the "channeling the counsel of elders" to licensed and formally trained homeopaths and other natural health practitioners.

To learn about this system, there are Bach Foundation approved courses taught in locations around the United States and also distance learning opportunities. There is also an endless supply of books written on the subject. I have listed a few of my favorites below.

The Bach Remedies Repertory by Wheeler
The Encyclopedia of Bach Flower Therapy by Scheffer (very thorough!)
Heal Thyself by Bach
Bach Flower Remedies by Bach
The Bach Remedies Workbook by Ball
Bach Flower Massage by Lo Rito

Healing and Belief

Carolyn Myss is one of the best known teachers
about the mind/body connection. This paper for my
Doctorate was based on one of her tapes:
Why People Don't Heal. [30]

One of Carolyn Myss' basic tenets is that your biography
becomes your biology. This is not a new concept and even
the ancients stated "as above, so below." Her belief (and I
agree with her) is that what we think and the life we live is
transferred into our bodies. We cannot separate the body and
mind or the body and spirit. There are new perceptions that
must be adopted. One is that we create our own reality. What
we think and believe happens to us. The second is that we
create our disease and therefore we can UNcreate our
disease. Most people don't want to hear this. It is much
easier to blame an unseen outside force rather than have to
take responsibility for our-selves, our thoughts and our lives.
I have seen numerous examples where what people think and
express becomes true. "I don't have enough money.", "My
back is killing me.", "This donut is going straight to my
hips." They have convinced themselves of those things and
their body is only too willing to oblige. What we think and
nurture in our minds is what happens; this is how our
biography becomes our biology.

In this society, healing can be extraordinarily
unattractive. We communicate and relate to others though
our pain and bad experiences. Saturday Night Live had a
whole skit, "Yesterday I stapled my tongue...oh I hate when
that happens." Then the two actors go on to top each other's
horrible experiences, all self-induced I might add.

---

[30] Myss, C. (2001). Why People Don't Heal – Recording. Boulder, CO:
Sounds True.

On the other side of the equation, most people don't want to know how great your life is and how healthy and wealthy you are. We feel bad sharing our successes with people who are down on their luck or unwell. If you hear for 30 minutes about your friend's failed marriage, crashed car, down stocks, dead cat, autistic child and back pain, it is socially unacceptable to then talk about how super your life is. Instead, we dig through our psyche to find something bad so we can relate and not seem like we're showing off. We feel guilt for our evolution.

At Christmas one year a relative asked how I was. I replied "amazing." With a disgusted face, she asked why I was amazing. I told her about my thriving business, my good health, my phenomenal husband and good grades and she dismissed me with a wave of the hand and a disinterested "uh huh." She then proceeded to tell another guest about how busy she had been, what a nightmare the kitchen remodel was and how sick she and the kids were (they are always, ALWAYS sick! A big surprise). She got a huge reaction and tons of attention for all the negativity and I received a grunt for my accomplishments.

We communicate those negative things through what Carolyn Myss calls "woundology." We bring up our past negative experiences so we can relate to others and/or have power over them. There are countless people who have met their mates at AA, suicide survivor groups, cancer therapy, etc. Right off the bat you know you are compatible as you are sharing the same wound. We yearn for connection to others in this society. If we can relate through pain and suffering, it becomes a bond that is hard to break. Certainly bad things happen to us, but we choose what story we tell and if we make something an anecdote or an identity. There are those people who obviously thrive on being a victim. Something is always going wrong, something is always a mess. They will call and tell you for hours about how bad everything is. Don't think about making a suggestion or offering a solution to their myriad problems, it wouldn't work because of *fill in the blank*. It becomes excuse after excuse of why their life is like it is and how it's not their fault. As the saying goes "misery loves company" and people bond through woundology. Myss says, "We agree to honor each other's wounds, and wounds equal power." It is much easier to hold court if you are suffering. Suffering equals power.

When I was 18 my mother passed away. She had been sick for many years and all my teachers knew that she was suffering and that I was understandably stressed out and upset. It was my senior year and being the typical over achiever, I was taking a full course load, plus directing a play, taking five dance classes, and acting in the school musical. There was one day that I was exhausted from all my activities and my teacher took me aside and said I was excused from the homework that week because I was obviously busy with my mom. I wasn't at all busy with my mom, I was busy with me. But I was not about to decline her offer of no homework for a week. And I began to realize that if I played the "sick mom card", I could get a lot of attention and a lot of special exceptions. I took advantage and life became really easy. I was also very conscious that I was doing it and I think most people do that without even knowing that they have mentioned for the 700th time that they were abused as a child and that is why they....drink, swear, are unhappy, etc.

I met a boy at my mother's funeral; he came because he had recently lost his father to cancer and wanted to comfort me. We started dating and talked a lot about how hard it was to lose a parent, etc. And soon we realized that we had nothing in common other than that experience and after we talked and cried, and talked some more and no more tears came, we had nothing else to do, so we broke up. I think most people stay in that frozen place and just keep crying and talking about the same old things. Eventually one person is done talking and wants to grow and it devastates the stuck person.

We have a friend who will not show his art in shows because 40 years ago a teacher criticized his work. Hundreds since have praised his work which inflates his ego, but he is listening to a three second comment from decades ago. He enjoys being stuck. No pressure, no failure, no risk, just a mean man from his youth. He is suffering from woundology and, his wound bank account is full.

Here are a few thoughts as to why people don't heal. (And there are certainly exceptions to what I am about to write, not everyone is like this.) We are not encouraged to take personal responsibility for things: our parents don't encourage it, our religions don't, and our government officials don't. It is best to blame some outside force for things that happen to us. If we take responsibility, then we become liable. We are to blame for our failings and our illnesses.

It is hard to be responsible; it involves risk and hurt and sacrifice. It's easier to blame the soviets, the terrorists, the Satanists, your parents, your teachers, God, whatever. When football players get a touchdown they thank God, when they miss a pass, they yell at the quarterback. Where does the player come into the equation?

If we return to Carolyn Myss' tenet of woundology, we see how habit forming the state of illness or a problematic life becomes. We get more attention in this society when things go wrong. If there is a group at a party and they are talking about life and someone takes a big sigh, head down, everyone suddenly wants to know what's wrong. And the person gets to hold court and gets hugs and pity and attention for the bad thing that just happened, or happened 20 years ago. It is a great excuse for not being present and not fulfilling your responsibilities. There is more reward for being stuck. Although most people believe they want to heal or improve their situation, on another level, they are addicted to their state of failure, sickness or other negative state. To truly heal means releasing this vision of yourself, and the attention it brings, and taking responsibility in your daily life for your actions, so you can grow and evolve. I don't think most people want to make that sacrifice.

"We fear change more than death", says Myss. I agree; change can be scary. But, it's also liberating. And it is through change that we grow. If you leave an abusive husband, that may also mean getting a job and being alone and not having the house and....not having that to complain about. It seems much easier to stay comfortably abused than be alone and in a state of personal responsibility.

Even if people want to heal, I think most people simply don't know how to start the process because we have never been taught what the process entails. They offer wood shop and home economics, math and science and English, but not communication, relationships and growth.

Though it is incredibly unhealthy to dwell on pain and relive a negative experience over and over again, the opposite, stuffing our feelings is just as unhealthy. Silently grasping onto painful experiences can be just as detrimental as those who talk about it constantly. I see people from my father's generation who simply will not talk about certain things. He will not discuss my mother's death and I suspect it still eats at him after 20 years. He speaks very little about his childhood or money, but is the first to tell a good dirty joke. A client of mine spoke briefly of her experience in Germany during the war. It was a fascinating, obviously difficult conversation for her. She has never told her children some of the things she shared with me. How long can we hold onto the pain that we suffered through? Obviously long enough that it makes us sick and unhappy. People find it so hard to forgive, themselves and others.

One way to learn from the past and move forward is to see a therapist. Yet for so many people, therapy is a taboo. They wouldn't dream of going because they perceive therapy as a weakness or as airing their dirty laundry in the square. They will quietly (or not so quietly) fester from the past.

I think it doesn't even occur to people that things can change. If they are prone to getting colds, it becomes their reality that they will catch whatever comes by. Or they can't ever read a map or can't ever do math. Whatever it is, how could it possibly change?

I never get sick. I tell people this frequently. They rarely ask me how I do it, but instead tell me how lucky I am and in turn, complain about how they are constantly sick. They attribute it to luck, which takes the power away from the individual with a healthy mind/body connection. Likewise, they perceive themselves as underlucky, another disempowering belief that self-perpetuates victimization and lack of personal responsibility. It doesn't even cross their minds that maybe they don't have to get sick either.

I also believe there is an overwhelming sense of fear: of change, of moving forward, of failing. Animals don't think about that. If the cheetah misses the first wildebeest, it doesn't go back to the pack and complain about the sun being its eyes, or that he didn't sleep well. The cheetah doesn't beat itself up over the failing. It runs and chases down the next herd. It is the key to survival and evolution. Humans can learn from the animals.

A client of mine said recently, "If you've got one foot in the past and one foot in the future, you end up pissing all over the present." And that is woundology and fear.

Healthy Pregnancy

Pregnancy is one of the most memorable times in a woman's life. You feel the joy and excitement of providing life for another. But along with that elation can come some not so pleasant side effects. Vomiting, nausea, swelling, acne, muscle and joint aches and mood swings are just some of the negative accompaniments to being pregnant. In many of these circumstances, Western medicine has little to contribute. However, complementary alternative medicine can offer assistance to enhance and ease pregnancy and labor. Here are a few natural additions that can help women during this very special time.

<u>Massage</u>

As a massage therapist that has worked on countless pregnant women, I can tell you the benefits are enormous. Massage can help with circulation, decreasing swelling in the hands and feet and relaxing the shoulders, low back and hip muscles. It also helps with carpal tunnel and tendinitis, which can flair up during pregnancy.[31] When searching for a prenatal massage, make sure the therapist is trained to work with expectant mothers. There are certain points on the body that should not be massaged during pregnancy, specifically some spots on the hands and feet.

Most pregnancy massage is performed with the woman on her side bolstered by pillows, but some therapists have special tables that accommodate bellies and breasts. As long as the mother feels okay to lie on her back, some of the session is done in that position as well. Make sure you communicate openly with the therapist about how you are feeling and if something is uncomfortable. Pregnant women

---

[31] http://www.pregnancytoday.com/articles/complications-in-pregnancy/carpal-tunnel-syndrome-and-pregnancy-1366/

can typically handle deeper massage, so have the therapist go as deep as you would like.

A great companion to massage is chiropractic. I am a big fan of this modality and during pregnancy it can be a great help for addressing body pain. Numerous sources say that more than half of all expectant mothers will experience low back pain at some point in the pregnancy. Between the postural changes and the weight gain (averaging 25-35 pounds)[32] it is no wonder that the body can feel uncomfortable. Chiropractic doctors specializing in pregnancy work specifically with the pelvis to restore balance. It helps with pelvis muscles, ligaments and can lead to a safer, quicker delivery.

"Chiropractic adjustments", says Dr. Crystal Clinton, a prenatal and pediatric chiropractor who specializes in the Webster Technique for pelvis stabilization, "reduce interference to the nervous system allowing your uterus to function at its maximum potential." And studies do show chiropractic adjustments reduce labor time.[33] Another bonus is that chiropractic can oftentimes turn around a breech birth, saving the mother a C-section.[34] If you want to try chiropractic, choose someone like Dr. Clinton that specializes in pregnancy. There are a few reasons not to get

---

[32] http://www.webmd.com/baby/guide/healthy-weight-gain

[33] Fallon, J. (1994). 25% lessening of labor time. Text Book on Chiropractic & Pregnancy. International Chiropractic Association, Virginia.

[34] Chiropractic Care: The late Larry Webster, D.C., of the International Chiropractic Pediatric Association, developed a technique which enabled chiropractors to release stress on the pregnant woman's pelvis and cause relaxation to the uterus and surrounding ligaments. The relaxed uterus would make it easier for a breech baby to turn naturally. The technique is known as the Webster Breech Technique.

The Journal of Manipulative and Physiological Therapeutics reported in the July/August 2002 issue that 82% of doctors using the Webster Technique reported success. Further, the results from the study suggest that it may be beneficial to perform the Webster Technique in the 8th month of pregnancy.

chiropractic such as bladder or bowel dysfunction, bleeding, cramping, faintness, and other symptoms and conditions. Check with your primary care provider if you have any questions.

Homeopathy

Most herbs are not recommended during pregnancy, but homeopathics are a safe and effective way to augment the body's natural systems. Steven Brynoff, ND, President of Mediral Homeopathics tells us that homeopathic remedies can work for "morning sickness, constipation, diarrhea, hemorrhoids and general circulation, pain and discomfort, insomnia, infections, incontinence, breech birth, late labor, slowing or speeding up labor, and exhaustion."

Homeopathy works on the principle that "like cures like." So if a large dose of a substance would cause certain symptoms, the homeopathic dosage of the same substance would eliminate those symptoms. By the time the homeopathic is consumed it contains no physical trace of the substance, just the essence. This is how you can take a dose of Arsenicum Album (white arsenic) and not get sick. In fact, a homeopathic dose of arsenic will treat the symptoms that mimic an arsenic overdose.

When working with homeopathics, it is best to choose a qualified practitioner. Since the remedies are chosen in response to each person's very specific symptoms, the premixed remedies available in health food stores may not be as effective as personalized treatment. Sandra Perko PhD says in her book *Homeopathy for the Modern Pregnant Woman and Her Infant*, "Homeopathy is the safest and most effective method of treatment in the pregnant woman's emotional and physical well-being." (See section on Homeopathics pg. 14 and Homeopathy for Children pg. 48)

Yoga

Yoga is a form of exercise that has become very main stream in our society. But did you know that you can continue your practice throughout your pregnancy? Prenatal yoga is available at private yoga studios and many gyms such as the YMCA. The benefits of prenatal yoga include increased strength, flexibility and well-being; reduced low back pain and sciatica; aided digestion; reduced swelling and fatigue in the joints.[35] Yoga helps ready the body for giving birth and improves emotional well-being. During the labor itself, yoga can help by preparing your body for breathing and introducing the concept of vocalization. Some yoga classes also incorporate visualization and meditation; this can be of enormous benefit if you are planning a drugless birth. Either way, yoga helps bond the body, mind and spirit to smooth the progress of labor.

Acupuncture

Acupuncture is not only well known for its help with fertility but can be used to enhance pregnancy and labor. It helps with nausea and vomiting, threatened miscarriage, heartburn, depression and babies in a breech position. Acupuncture has been shown to help ripen the cervix and reduce labor time. When looking for a practitioner, check to see if they have a background in women's health or labor and delivery.[36]

Doula

What the heck is a doula? A doula is an assistant that is present for the mother and her partner during pregnancy and labor. Some people think their spouse or companion will be enough support, but it can't hurt to have another person with you, stroking your hair, massaging your feet and translating what the doctors and nurses just said to you. Studies have shown that having a doula decreases the length

---

[35] http://www.expectantmothersguide.com/library/cleveland/benefits-of-prenatal-yoga.htm and other numerous sources on line.

[36] http://www.acufinder.com/Acupuncture+Information/Detail/ACUPUNCTURE+AND+PREGNANCY

of labor by 25%, decreases cesarean births by 50%, and reduces need for epidurals, forceps, narcotics and pitocin.[37]

I feel my role as a birth assistant is to support the mother and her companion and make sure her birth plan is followed. I offer support with homeopathics, Reiki, massage, encouraging words, relieving the partner so he/she can rest, aromatherapy and anything else the mother could need. I have even taken video and photos. Labor can be very emotional for the family members present and having an impartial person like a doula or birth assistant can be a huge help to everyone present.

I hope this quick overview will help you make informed choices about your pregnancy. Good luck!

---

[37] Klaus, MH, Kennell, JH, Klaus, PH. (1993). Compiled from Mothering the Mother. Addison Wesley Publishing Co.

Homeopathy for Children

It seems that no matter what time of year it is, kids are bringing home every cold, flu and ailment they come across. Antibiotics, flu shots and over-the-counter medications are certainly options, but what about an alternative solution that has been around for 200 years? Homeopathics have been used for centuries to treat ailments and illnesses with great success, with no side effects. They are easy to give to children and can be very effective for illness such as earaches, colds and sore throats. But the first question; what the heck is homeopathy?

Homeopathy works on the principle of "like cures like." Giving someone a minute dose of a substance will cause the body to eliminate symptoms that in a large dose would cause those same symptoms. (For example, a big dose would cause a fever; a homeopathic dose would eliminate the fever.) This teeny-weeny amount of a substance jump starts the body's own defenses to act on the problem. Let's look at the principles of Classical Homeopathy.

Classical Homeopathy involves comprehensive questioning and analysis of a patient's symptoms and physical, emotional and spiritual responses to each disorder. For example, a headache would be examined in regards to: what brought it on, what makes it better or worse, is there a time of day that aggravates it, is it limited to a certain part of the head, what were the circumstances that caused it, etc. After assessing that information a remedy would be chosen. And, although two people may both have a headache, they will most likely have very different answers to those questions, and thus be prescribed two different remedies. In Western medicine, it is the same headache. Classical homeopathy is used most often to treat a specific disease or symptom like stomachache or sore throat.

The Benefits of Homeopathics:

- Homeopathy is not a "one size fits all" system of medicine like we see in most Western modalities. This is individualized medicine exclusive to each patient.

- Physical disease can be treated as well as emotional and spiritual issues; symptoms are not just covered up.

- There are no adverse side effects as there can be with prescription or over the counter (OTC) medication, thus it is totally appropriate for children, pregnant women and even pets.

- Another benefit is the affordability of the substances. Homeopathics are VERY inexpensive, typically $5-$7 per remedy.

- Use of homeopathics can produce lasting change in the body. It is not a temporary relief of symptoms; it helps the body truly heal itself.

Working with homeopathics for your family:

First I suggest writing down everything that is going on with the illness. Here are some things you will want to know:

How did it start? Gradually, suddenly, after exposure to cold, etc.

Where does it hurt, specifically? Not just, "my head hurts", but what part of the head? The more detailed the better.

What does it feel like? Is it heavy, scratchy, burning, itchy; is it on one side of the body more than the other? Once again, the more descriptors the better.

Is there discharge? What does it look like? Is it copious? Watery? Yellow? Discharge is an important key to what the body is doing and helps you find a remedy.

What personality signs are showing with the illness? Is the child suddenly clingy, angry, or pouty? Note what behaviors are different than normal.

Is there anything bizarre? Does the child have irregular cravings, like an extreme desire for cold liquids, or exhibit strange behavior, like crying until put in a bath tub? In homeopathy, sometimes the most bizarre symptom is the one that clues you in to the right remedy.

Now that you have written all that down, you need to find the right remedy. There are great pediatric homeopathy books on the market that key you in to the right remedy, and there are also remedy finders on line. I like the books *Everybody's Guide to Homeopathic Medicines* by Cummings and Ullman, *Homeopathic Medicine for Children and Infants* by Ullman, or *The Spirit of Homeopathic Medicines* by Didier Grandgeorge. There are sections for children and also most adult ailments and they give you ideas of what information you will need for each symptom. Once you find the right remedy, head to your local health food store and buy it. They are very affordable and because you use so little of it, it can last a long time.

Here is an example for you. A child comes home with an ear ache. He is craving physical contact and wants to be held. He wants fresh air, is not thirsty at all and there is yellow discharge from the ear and nose. This leads to the remedy **Pulsatilla**. Another child is in the later stages of the earache. She's weak, tired and whimpers but is not as interested in physical contact. She's chilly and likes being under warm blankets but her hands, feet and head are sweaty. The remedy for her would be **Silica**. (I found this information in *Everybody's Guide to Homeopathic Medications*, mentioned above.)

If this sounds too complicated for you there are other options. One is to consult a homeopathic practitioner in your area. They will take down the signs and symptoms and give you the right remedy. Another option is to use a combination remedy that is available in most health food stores.

Companies take the most common remedies for any given ailment, combine them all together and sell them that way. They have combination remedies for everything from teething to PMS. A combination remedy I recommend for the flu is Oscillococcinum; it works best when you feel the first hint that illness is coming on. Homeopathics are available in sugar tablets, lactose tablets and liquids. They are all just as effective; just choose the one that works for you or is most readily available. Your health food store professional can point you in the right direction and often they have books available there that you can look through.

(Just a side note: If you buy an individual remedy based on your research, don't worry about the one or two disorders it has listed on the label. They just write some of the most common; it doesn't mean you can't use it for other things)

I encourage you to explore this classical system of medicine and experiment to see if it might help you and your family.

Recommended Books:

Homeopathic Medicine at Home by Dana Ullman, MPH. 1992.

The Spirit of Homeopathic Medicines by Didier Grandgeorge. 1998.

Everybody's Guide to Homeopathic Medicines by Cummings and Ullman. 1997.

Even Wonder Woman Needs a Day Off: Dealing with Stress

We are living in a phenomenal time when women can be the breadwinners and the dinner makers, the mothers and the CEOs. No longer are we relegated to nurses, teachers and barefoot and pregnant. What else comes with these opportunities? Pressure, anxiety, over-work and too much responsibility. We are taking on the world and its stresses as well. In this high-powered woman world, here are some low key stress busters. It is important to take care of business, but it's even more important to take care of ourselves. No time? Think again!

<u>Slow Food</u>:

How many times have we rushed out of the house and shoved something stale and packaged into our mouths?

- Keep healthy food in your car, in your desk and in your cupboards. Bars and nuts are great snacks and can be a full meal if necessary. I love Cavewoman bars, they are all natural. You can find them at <u>www.cavewomanbars.com</u>.

- Make sure you drink enough water, not soda which is one of the unhealthiest things you can consume. And if you are stressed, the last thing you need is caffeine and sugar which may cause a crash later.

- Eat slowly - preferably not in your car, during an argument or in front of the depressing news or a violent TV show. Stress slows the digestive system and eating under duress can wreak havoc with your stomach and intestines.

- Chew…a lot (grandma was right!), and try to make sure your diet is balanced with lots of fresh veggies.

One a day:

Stressed women need extra vitamins and minerals, especially taking into account various times of the month and menopause.

- I suggest everyone take a high quality vitamin, mineral and amino acid supplement.

- The B vitamins are great at helping with stress, depression and sleep, but take them earlier in the day as they can cause disruption of sleep if taken too late.

- Anti-oxidants like C, E, and selenium are important to help fight the aging that extra stress causes.

- Calcium and magnesium are especially important for women. Magnesium can help with PMS, headaches and menstrual cramps.

- Homeopathic remedies, Bach Flower Essences and Acupuncture can be great for helping to cope with stress. (See pages 33 for more detail on Bach Flowers and 14 on Homepathics)

To sleep perchance to catch up!

Lack of sleep has been linked with obesity, depression and shorter life span.[38], [39] There are numerous healthy sleep suggestions:

- Don't do anything in bed other than sleep (Well, sex is okay too and a great stress buster). See page 81 for more sleep info.

---

[38] http://archive.mailtribune.com/archive/2006/1024/life/stories/sleep-main.htm

[39] http://therapyforsleep.com/index.cfm/fuseaction/main.affects/sleepAffectsEveryPartofYourLife.html

- If you have trouble falling asleep, supplements like Melatonin, Valerian Root or L-Tryptophan can help as well as homeopathics like Moondrops by Historical Remedies (www.historicalremedies.com).

- Keep a notebook by the bed so if you wake in the night remembering that you have to do something, you can do a mind-dump and get it out. Don't dwell.

- Don't eat or drink too late in the day as that can affect your sleep. Most people think alcohol will relax them. It is a stimulant at first, but with prolonged consumption it may cause sleeplessness and dehydration.

- Try to go to sleep early and wake with the sun. Don't nap as that can throw off your circadian rhythms.

The 3 Rs. Relax. Relax. Relax

- Breathe and try yoga, tai chi or chi gong, or other relaxing practices that exercise the mind and body.

- Pay attention to your posture. Holding your shoulders up or your neck tight keeps your stress level higher and your muscles tense.

- Meditate. Still your mind and go inside to a quiet place of comfort and stability. Many people think they aren't good at meditating. Don't strive for perfection, just retreat inside.

A+.

Remember it is not the amount of stress. It's how you deal with the stress. I'm a type A personality. Because of this I am more prone to heart issues, stress related disease and stroke. (Great! Productive and on schedule, but dead.)

I know my limits, but the problem comes when something unexpected pushes those limits. These unplanned distractions increase our negative reaction to stress. If you create a buffer, then you are better equipped to deal with an unplanned event, rather than if you schedule everything down to the millisecond.

It's That Time

Many women have trouble with PMS. That's a subject that could fill its own book but I wanted to touch on some solutions here.

- Diet matters. Eliminate sugar, caffeine and dairy, and reduce eggs and meat, as these aggravate PMS in many women. Add magnesium as it helps with cramps, headaches and PMS. Take Omega 3 fatty acids. The herb Black Cohosh can be taken as a preventative. Make sure you are getting enough exercise also.

- Emotions. It is believed that the PMS symptoms we have are illustrating unbalance in our life. Studies show that women who are codependent or have alcoholics in their lives are more prone to PMS. Take this time every month to examine your relationships and your feelings about those around you. Get in touch, express your feelings and see if your symptoms don't subside.

So ladies, my successful and marvelous friends; take a deep breath, get your shoulders back down where they should be and realize that no matter how much we accomplish, it doesn't matter if we are too unhealthy and busy to enjoy it! And now I'm going to set down my golden lariat, take off my bullet proof bracelets and relax on Paradise Isle with the other powerful women!

Home Care

Nothing beats a day at the spa; relaxing environment, facial, pedicure, good deep tissue massage, a tinkling fountain and ambient music. But in this economic environment, an expensive day out might not be on the top of your list. What can you do at home to keep your health and relaxation at its peak? Here are a few suggestions.

Soak your cares away

Nothing says relaxation like a hot bath and a good book. For achy muscles, use inexpensive Epsom salts available at most drug and health food stores. These mainly consist of the mineral magnesium, which has been shown to relax muscles and flush toxins. Add a scented bath oil or bubble bath for aromatherapy enhancement, but remember to choose natural or organic products whenever possible, as bath time should not be about inhaling and soaking in chemicals found in mainstream beauty and bath products.

If you don't have a tub, some gyms and YMCAs will offer day passes, most of which include a jacuzzi or hot tub. This is an affordable way to "take the waters."

Table talk

Just because it's dinner at home for you and your spouse, or you alone, doesn't mean it has to be paper napkins and the "everyday" plates. Light some candles, use the good silver and crystal and enjoy your meal at home like it was a five-star dinner out. Try a new recipe, make up a menu and serve it professionally. It can be fun to try out new foods and make it feel like luxury dining in the comfort of your own kitchen.

Pamper party

Invite a few girlfriends over and take turns treating each other to manicures and pedicures. This is a great way to relax and bond, and try out new shades of polish. You can also do the same thing with mini-facials. Beauty supply stores and most drug stores sell home face scrubs, masks and toners. I personally love Burt's Bees products. Have everyone bring their favorite product and make it a pot-luck lunch. Experiment with what you like and treat your galpals to an affordable day of beauty at your place.

Rub me the right way

There are plenty of massage tools on the market that are specifically for self-care. When working with massage tools, use care in trying them out on other people. Since you can't feel the tissue, you have a greater chance of hurting them. A good rule of thumb is to try the massage tools on yourself first, so you can gauge appropriate pressure. When in doubt, a simple and effective massage tool is a golf or tennis ball. Place the ball beneath the area of tension and use your body weight to roll around on it.

If you want to do a full body massage on your partner, light some candles, put on some soft music, break out the massage oil and rub away! If you're not sure what to do or are afraid of hurting yourself or them, I have a new instructional DVD that can teach the basics of safe and effective massage at home. It can be found on my website: www.healingcirclemassage.com/instructional_dvd and is also a perfect gift!

Work those muscles

Sometimes it's hard to get motivated to exercise, especially at home and not in the normal "gym" environment. This is a good time to turn your housework into fitness. Do lunges while you vacuum and curls with your groceries. When relaxing for the night in front of the TV, sit on the floor and stretch. See if you can make it through a whole block of commercials doing sit ups or crunches. Sometimes these little tricks can keep us going. It is so important to use your body. Take this little bit of time everyday for your health. You and your body will appreciate it!

Tea'd off

How about organizing a high tea for your friends? Have everyone wear an outrageous hat, cut the crusts off some cucumber sandwiches and balance little plates on your lap. Ask everyone to try out a British accent. Give a prize for the craziest hat or best/worst accent. Organizing theme parties like this at home can be a great way to reconnect with friends or meet new friends of friends. Parties don't have to cost a lot money and you don't have to leave the house to have a good time.

Playing around

Invite everyone you know for a game night. Have your guests bring their favorite board game, have a few card tables set up and play the night away. This is a great way to cut loose, relax and pretend you're a kid again. Why shouldn't grown ups have play dates too?

Whatever you choose to do at home, make your relaxation frequent and your health a priority!

Introduction to Corporate Health

This article first appeared in the Pacific Coast Business Times
and is the first in a series on Corporate Health

In my 20 years of therapeutic massage and natural health experience I have treated injuries ranging from torn rotator cuffs to whiplash and sciatica. What I see increasing on my table are repetitive stress injuries like carpal tunnel syndrome. I am noticing that my desk job clients are coming in more beat up than my extreme athletes. What is causing this increase and what can be done about it? I intend to educate people in the office before they end up on my table or under the doctor's knife. It can be done; it just takes some dedication and education. In this series of articles I'm going to tell you how to be healthier at work, not just physically but all aspects of wellness. We will talk about things like stretching, taking breaks, nutrition and tips on how to fit it all in to your busy day. You and your co-workers will learn how to be a healthier office!

More and more companies are talking about corporate wellness. But what exactly does that mean and how can it help your business? With the high cost of health care, the ramifications of injured employees and the risk of Workers Compensation claims; many corporations are instituting policies to encourage better health. Whether it is chair massage, gym memberships, yoga, stretching or ergonomic consultations, companies are becoming proactive in keeping their staff healthy and well.

According to the National Institute of Occupational Safety and Health, repetitive stress injuries are now the single largest cause of occupational health problems in the U.S.,[40] with a quarter of workers in occupations that can

---

[40] http://www.cdc.gov/niosh/updates/ergprs.html

cause repetitive stress injuries (RSI). So, it is in the best interest of the company to keep everyone safe.

Carpal tunnel and tendonitis can be avoided with proper posture, stretching, breaks, nutrition and station set up. We can't just blame ergonomics for these problems though. Forty years ago, secretaries didn't have the latest contoured chair or a consultant measuring how far their typewriter was from their eyes. They varied their activities and even if their day was composed of just typing, they had to wind the tape, roll the paper, make corrections, etc. Now with the word processor, we can type for hours, never having to change positions or move at all. We have convenienced ourselves into a state of injury. And the smaller the gadgets get, the harder it is on our arms and eyes. Blackberrys, I-phones and PDAs are contributing to finger and wrist issues. I know we need to use them, but counter that activity by putting them down occasionally and stretching.

We cannot hold technology solely responsible for these problems either; employees have to be conscious about their bodies and their health. Many staff work too long in one position without stopping. By law, breaks are provided but I know many who don't take them. In many cases there are imposed deadlines, too little staff and too much work. We have to find the balance between productivity and our own well-being.

It is also common to find people eating poor quality food at their desks or never taking a break to walk around or go to the bathroom, let alone stretch and exercise. It is important that we listen to our body's cues and stop when we need to (every 50 minutes or so is ideal). It benefits everyone in the long run to take time to stretch, eat a nutritious meal or snack and walk around in the sun for just five minutes.

And once the work day is over, it is important to stay active and fit. Working on the computer all day and then going home to play computer games is problematic from a health perspective. Management can't control what staff does outside the office, but logic dictates this isn't the best choice. Try to find hobbies that use different parts than those you are already overusing at work. Data entry people who go home and knit, garden and do beading are just asking for hand issues. And often times it becomes a Workers Comp problem. It is time for us all to take responsibility for ourselves and our wellness. Stretch, eat right and exercise. I will teach you how to do all these things and more.

This has been a tough year economically and the companies that have survived are starting to feel the pressure to keep their remaining employees happy. Letting your staff know that you care about their wellbeing and health is a way to ensure better productivity and loyalty. We will look at ways to encourage better office health and I will give you tips and hints to fit in fitness, revamp your kitchen to provide healthier foods, and stretches and exercises that can be easily incorporated into your day. Until next time, have a healthy day!

For more information about Healthier Office, check out www.healthieroffice.com.

10 Quick Health Tips

1. Take a break

It is recommended that you get up and move around every 50 minutes to an hour. Most people rush through their day, eating at their desk, never leaving their work station. That can lead to repetitive stress injuries and job burn out. Make it a point to stretch and move at various times throughout the day. When you head to the bathroom, take a few extra minutes to move your body. Or while waiting for something to print, use that as YOUR time.

2. Men, low back or hip pain?

Many men come to my office with these complaints, and as they turn to go into the treatment room I see a large protrusion on one butt cheek. It's not a tumor, it's a wallet! And when you sit on it consistently, it can throw your whole body out of alignment. We are designed to be symmetrical and our body will compensate to make that happen. So keep your wallet elsewhere! Women, be ware of a heavy purse. It can pull your shoulders out of alignment and cause upper back and neck pain.

3. Supplements

No matter how much "good food" we consume, we are just not getting the nutrients we require. Add to that all the processed foods that make their way into our diets and it becomes clear that we need to supplement. A multi-vitamin and mineral formula keeps our body functioning properly and can curb food cravings. Amino acids are also an important supplement, as there are many amino acids we cannot produce ourselves, that are nonetheless needed for processes in the body.

4. Lay off the Soda

Diet <u>or</u> regular, soda is just plain bad for you. Regular soda contains high fructose corn syrup which is shown to be linked to the epidemics of obesity and type-2 diabetes.[41] Diet soda contains artificial sweetener, which has been associated with numerous health problems. Both diet and regular soda have high amounts of phosphorus, which can interfere with calcium absorption and contribute to osteoporosis and heart disease.

5. Good Bacteria

If you have ever taken any antibiotics or have bowel issues such as diverticulitis or Irritable Bowel Syndrome (IBS) you might be low on good bacteria in the colon, which is needed for elimination. The bacteria also produce many necessary vitamins like the Bs. Make sure you take live Probiotics with at least 60 billion CFUs (colony forming units).

6. Spring Cleaning

Some alternative medicine practitioners believe that we have between five and 15 pounds of feces in our colon. That does NOT lead to good health. Cleansing and fasting can help move that along. When a person fasts the body begins a process of cleansing and repairing. Most colon hydro therapists recommend regular fasting to enhance the immune system and strengthen the body. It is a good idea to cleanse at least seasonally, with colon hydrotherapy recommended. Cleansing is not just for a sick body. Everyone can benefit from cleansing and fasting.

Let's talk briefly about transit time. Dr. Jensen in his book on bowel care and other experts say that our food

---

[41] American Chemical Society (2007, August 23) Soda Warning? High-fructose Corn Syrup Linked to Diabetes, New Study Suggests. ScienceDaily. http://www.sciencedaily.com/releases/2007/08/070823094819.htm

should move through us in 18 hours.[42] You can check this by eating beets, unshelled sunflower seeds or corn. If your transit time is too fast you might not be getting all the nutrients you need and if it is too slow, food might be putrefying in your system and causing other issues.

7. Exercise

We all know we should exercise regularly, but exercise can help with things you never suspected like good bowel function. Leslie Shinkle, an ACE certified instructor reminds us that "exercise boosts our self-confidence and allows us to perform daily tasks easier." Even housework can help. Leslie recommends adding lunges while you vacuum or curls while you carry your groceries. "Anything to get you off the couch and moving is a positive step towards health."

8. Adjustments

Chiropractic is obviously good for structural issues such as whiplash and sciatica. But Dr. John Craviotto with 25 years chiropractic experience reminds us that other disorders can be helped through adjustments. "Keeping the spine aligned keeps the nervous system functioning at 100%. That helps our immune system and assists us in fighting disease."

Feel chiropractic is a scam? Dr Craviotto responds, "A racket is when the same treatment plan is prescribed for everyone regardless of what they need. Some people with chronic problems do need to be seen for six months; other people only need to be seen once or twice. The main issue is, is there improvement? You have to trust your chiropractor, just as you do your doctor and your mechanic. If you don't...find someone else."

---

[42] Jensen, Bernard Dr., (1999). Dr. Jensen's Guide to Better Bowel Care. Pg. 2. Avery Publishing.

9. Rx

Many people take prescriptions. Often, prescription drugs have side effects that lead to other prescriptions. Issues such as insomnia, sleepiness, headaches and muscle aches can be side effects. This phenomenon is known as iatrogenic disease. Know your medication and if what you are taking could be causing your new problem. And just because you have been on a medication for a long time, doesn't mean it couldn't be the culprit. www.webmd.com is a great resource. If you suspect that your current prescriptions might be causing new side effects, discuss your symptoms and concerns with your doctor.

10. Go East

Traditional Chinese medicine (TCM) can be a great form of maintenance. It is recommended to do acupuncture when you know you are susceptible to ailments. If you know a certain time of year or season change is a problem for you with things like allergies, bronchitis, etc., acupuncture can help with those transitions. Acupuncture is also beneficial for overall health promotion and conditions like indigestion, insomnia, headaches, colds, PMS, depression and even smoking cessation.

If you have never had acupuncture, give it a shot; it is virtually painless and can help balance the system and promote overall health and wellness.

Obesity and Natural Health

You can't watch the news or a read a magazine without some chatter about the obesity epidemic in the US. It's true we are fatter than ever, and millions of dollars are being spent on diets, pills, obesity-related illness and weight reduction surgeries. If you are struggling with your weight, what can you do? There are so many factors contributing to weight gain that it can be overwhelming. However, there are many things you can do to lose that weight and this article gives you some of those options.

First off, I want to explain leptin and its impact on our eating patterns. Leptin is a chemical in the brain that tells us when we are full. Some of us have more leptin than others and the higher the leptin, the faster you realize you are full. It has also been discovered that artificial sweeteners like aspartame actually suppress leptin. This is particularly frustrating for weight conscious individuals, as artificial sweeteners are frequently used in diet products. So in a way, the leptin suppressing diet products become self defeating as no matter how much of these foods and beverages you consume, you won't feel full and will want to keep eating. This is why I recommend doing away with pre-packaged foods, "diet" products, artificial sweeteners or soda.

Soda

Neither diet nor regular soda have any nutritional value and can be a contributing factor to weight gain. In fact, multiple studies have found correlations between high fructose corn syrup (found in non-diet soda and many processed foods) and weight gain in this country. [43], [44]

---

[43] http://seattletimes.nwsource.com/html/health/2002658491_healthsyrup04.html

Though some scientists refute these claims, I still avoid products with high fructose corn syrup as it has no nutritional value and why risk it if it does indeed cause weight gain?

Alcohol

I also recommend cutting back on alcohol. Although wine certainly has been shown to have health benefits it is an empty calorie beverage. And since the body burns alcohol before fat, it might leave you happy but chunky.

Water

Drinking enough water is vital for weight loss. Make sure you're getting at least the 8 recommended glasses per day. It not only keeps you hydrated, but is a calorie free way to fill your stomach and give you a sense of fullness.

Vegetables First

I also suggest starting every meal with a big salad or helping of vegetables. They are rich in necessary minerals, a great source of fiber and are very filling. You won't be as likely to overeat if you start with healthy vegetables. And eat slowly. Give your brain a chance to realize you're full and signal you to stop eating.

Healthy Fats

When it comes to weight loss and food, there is no one size fits all approach. Some people do better cutting out carbs, others benefit from cutting out fat. Remember though, we do need SOME fat as it is essential for healthy hair, skin, muscles, and brain function and helps metabolize certain vitamins. Make sure however, that you are getting healthy fats, like olive oil, avocado, flax seed oil, etc. What you

---

[44] Bray, G., Nielsen, S., Popkin, B. Consumption of high-fructose corn syrup in beverages may play a role in the epidemic of obesity. American Journal of Clinical Nutrition, Vol. 79, No. 4, 537-543, April 2004.

should be avoiding at all costs is Trans Fat. These come from hydrogenated or partially hydrogenated oils. Even if a packages states "no trans fats" if there is any hydrogenated or partially hydrogenated oils in the ingredients, it has Trans Fats in it. Let's stick with real food that our grandparents ate; if my 82 year old grandmother never heard of it, I try to avoid eating it.

Diets

There are many diet plans that encourage elimination of carbohydrates. Again this works for only a certain percentage of the population. South Beach Diet and Atkins are two programs that do away with carbs. I caution anyone starting a carb limiting diet to be aware that they are geared toward a lifetime change in diet, not a temporary fix. If you are going to do a diet plan, make sure it's something you can stick with forever.

I have many clients that have had success with Weight Watchers - it's not only easy to follow, but you get the support of a group environment. Having people in your life cheer you on and not sabotage you is very important for a weight loss plan. This is especially important if your partner is not supportive due to fears of how a big change in you will affect the relationship or if they have struggled with weight loss themselves.

Chemical Calories

There is a new buzz in the science community about something called chemical calories. We have been seeing evidence that pesticides, herbicides and plastics are accumulating in our fat cells and may affect the body's ability to burn fat. Our bodies are not designed to handle these artificial components. Many of the animals we consume for food have been given chemicals to fatten them quickly; these chemicals might also be fattening us. These pervasive toxins have also been shown to damage our weight control system. For more information about chemical calories I recommend the book *The Body Restoration Plan* by Paula Baillie-Hamilton.

Prescription Side Effects

Some prescription drugs like steroids and antidepressants may also have the side effect of weight gain. Some people's bodies are better at shedding these toxic compounds than others. To help remove these compounds from our bodies, it might be useful to do a cleanse or a fast. Be careful not to fast too fast though as the toxins can mobilize too rapidly and cause us to get ill. Start slowly and consult a dietician or physician for help.

Watch Those Portions

As the movie *Supersize Me* points out, America's food portions have gotten out of control. Our food is not only worse than it was 20 years ago, but we're consuming more of it. The "clean your plate" generation is getting bigger and bigger. Combine that with clever marketing and cartoon characters selling bad food and our children are bearing the brunt of the weight problem. According to the Center for Disease Control, 11-18% of our children are overweight depending on age and this seems to be increasing as time goes on.[45] It's critical to start good food education early and try to encourage kids to eat healthy and exercise more.

Exercise

It used to be thought that the key to losing weight was as easy as balancing calories in with calories out. This equation certainly does make a difference, and we have to exercise to burn calories. We all have a unique resting metabolism that varies among people, but moving our bodies, working up a sweat and finding exercise that we enjoy is extraordinarily important to weight loss. The key is finding something that YOU like to do, not what your

[45] http://www.cdc.gov/nchs/fastats/overwt.htm

neighbor or husband enjoys, but that YOU enjoy. If exercise is a problem for you because of your weight or joint problems, look into low impact exercise like a recumbent bike or water aerobics. It's a great start to get you active.

Herbal Supplements

Let's talk briefly about supplements. There have been diet pills as long as people have consumed food. Be ware of ads that promise too much. To be able to "Drop 30 pounds overnight with no exercise" may sound great, but what will this do to your body? And is it really possible? The pounds came on one at a time over many years and they must go off the same way. Unfortunately there is no magic pill, but there are a few herbal supplements that will be safer on the body. Chromium has been used for years to help with diabetes. It also allegedly speeds up metabolism. When taken with HCA (Hydroxycitric acid) it showed slowing of the appetite and decreased fat stores in recent studies. [46] 5HTP which is a precursor to serotonin in the brain helped women feel fuller sooner and consume less carbs. It also showed lowering of blood glucose levels. [47] This supplement is also great for addressing depression and aiding sleep (do not take 5HTP if you are on SSRIs for depression). Caffeine is a metabolism booster and green tea extract is recommended as a healthy source.

We often look at heavier people and assume they got that way purely by eating too much bad food, but that's not always the case. As mentioned before, low production of leptin, chemical calories or prescription side effects could be the culprit. There are other hidden causes of weight gain.

- Thyroid insufficiency and adrenal fatigue can contribute to weight gain; have a blood test to check your

[46] http://web.winltd.com/Article.aspx?PageURL=/Pages/English/health news/synergisticpartners.htm

[47] http://www.ideamarketers.com/library/printarticle.cfm? articleid=416729

hormone levels. If you are having trouble with sleep, mood, temperature and a thinning of your eyebrows, you might be hypothyroid. Consult your physician. Be aware that the normal range for thyroid function is very vast; you may be within "normal" range and still be hypothyroid. Talk to your doctor if you are having symptoms but test normal.

- Stress, which releases cortisol in the body is now being linked to belly fat. Relax more!

- Heredity, which we can only do so much about, can also be a link to obesity. On the other hand, I believe we are in control of our lives and in some instances, can overcome heredity issues. Sometimes it's an easy out to say, "Well, my whole family is big." You might not have to carry on the tradition; try to make a different choice.

- Depression: Scientists are seeing links between depression and obesity. Quite often when people are depressed they tend to eat more and exercise less. If you are feeling depressed see a professional. They can help you manage your depression from multiple angles.

- Lack of Sleep: Studies have also shown that lack of sleep can contribute to inability to lose weight. Make sure you're getting your zzzz's.

Goal Setting

I want to conclude with goal setting. Make sure your goals are realistic. We have a set point of body weight that our bodies try to maintain. This is different for everyone. We can't change it! For our natural set point to work properly, we must have proper nutrients, exercise, an intact brain and proper hormone balance. I see many people aiming for a weight or body size that they are never going to reach. Don't idolize models and celebrities; they have the time and money for trainers, custom food and airbrushing. Try not to compare yourself to others around you. We should be striving to be healthy in our own bodies, regardless of our current size. Yes, extra weight has social stigma and leads to illness, but the important thing should be health not looks. Set realistic goals and know that achieving long term weight loss is a time commitment, but the rewards are truly worth it. Good luck in your journey!

Energy Boosters

We've all observed children playing. We watch for a second and then say, "Gee, I wish I had their energy." And then everyone laughs as they remember what it was like to not tire as quickly as we do now. I am not guaranteeing you'll be running around the playground by morning, but I do have some suggestions that can help boost your energy.

Nutritional Supplements

Proper nutrition is key to energy levels. Since most of the food we eat is either processed, irradiated, minerally depleted, genetically modified, sprayed with a chemical, or artificial, I recommend taking a high quality vitamin and mineral supplement. The B vitamins are essential for good energy. Increasing B6 and B12 is my first suggestion for weary clients. Don't take them too late in the day though, or they may disrupt your sleep.

Getting a wide variety of minerals is also essential. Everyone stresses the importance of calcium, but there are so many more minerals we need like iron, magnesium, molybdenum, copper, zinc, etc. Taking a good multi mineral supplement can help. Also remember that we need protein for energy. Amino acids, which are the building blocks of protein, can be taken in supplement form. I especially recommend this for vegetarians or non-red meat eaters.

Sweeteners

When we hit that afternoon slump, most people reach for the soda or candy bar. We use glucose as an energy source so often we crave something sweet. Make sure that what you're eating contains real sugar and not high fructose corn syrup or some artificial sweetener. These trick our bodies into thinking we are getting sugar but it's really an unusable substance. Whole food snacks like fruits, dates and juices contain natural sugars. Don't over do it on the sugar though, or you will crash later and feel worse.

Ginseng

Ginseng is a natural stimulant that can be taken in herbal form or can be found in specialty beverages. Make sure what you are drinking actually has ginseng and not just a high amount of caffeine. Too much ginseng, like caffeine, can cause a racing heart, palpitations or nervousness. Again, moderation is the key. And speaking of caffeine, I personally don't believe caffeine is bad if consumed in moderation. Though remember, drowsiness is not a caffeine deficiency! Too much can cause sleep disturbances, jitteriness, heart issues, anxiety and is often addictive. Ever have that day where you can't get your morning java? How long before that headache kicks in? Try not to have caffeine too late in the day as it might interrupt your sleep. Of if you're prone to heart issues or anxiety, consider eliminating it all together.

Beware of Energy Drinks

The newest boosting craze are energy drinks like Red Bull, No Fear, Full Throttle and Rockstar. These drinks are high in sugar and caffeine and can lead to a later crash and physical addiction. This is much worse for children than adults. High amounts of caffeine cause extra excretion of calcium, which in young girls can lead to adult onset of osteoporosis. These drinks can also be very addicting.

Another new trend is mixing these energy drinks with alcohol. From a health standpoint, this is a dangerous combination. Alcohol is a depressant and caffeine and sugar are stimulants. Yes, it allows you to drink more alcohol but this combination could be disastrous as it clouds your judgment as to how drunk you actually are. This can lead to driving with someone intoxicated, taking sexual risks and increased injury.

Exercise

I know the last thing you want to do when you are already tired is exercise, but studies consistently show that exercise can actually boost your energy levels. In fact, a recent review of twelve large-scale studies on the connection between exercise and fatigue concluded that all studies found a direct link between physical activity and reduced fatigue for participants who were physically active compared to those who were inactive. Other research shows that even among people with chronic illness like cancer or heart disease, exercise can ward off feelings of fatigue and help people feel more energized. This doesn't mean you have to run five miles. Even 15-20 minutes of walking or light exercise can make a difference.

Stay Hydrated

Since our bodies are 80% water, it is important to keep yourself hydrated. If we wait until we feel the sensation of thirst, it is too late; we're already dehydrated. Drink water throughout the day which helps with blood flow and removal of toxins. Remember caffeine is a diuretic, which causes increased output of urine, so caffeinated drinks don't count. Pure water is the best!

Deep Breathing

We can also boost energy by deep breathing. Oxygen carries energy to our cells which will give us a natural perk. Try four slow deep breaths, (use your abdomen not just your chest) and get a natural high.

Get Enough Sleep

It stands to reason that if you are not sleeping well, you are going to have low energy the next day. It's a myth that we need eight hours of sleep. We need as much as we need. Some people are fine on six hours, others need nine or ten. Go to bed when you are tired if at all possible. Don't force yourself to stay awake at night, especially by artificial means. And during the day, if you're really tired and can take a nap, take one. But make it short. Don't sleep too much or you will have trouble sleeping that night.

Attitude Makes a Difference

If we are constantly telling ourselves that we're tired and have no energy, we are just programming the body to behave that way. Change your mind to change your body. Try affirmations like: "I am well-rested and energized." "I am filled with vigor." "My energy is boundless." You will have better results with positive thinking.

If you are finding that your energy is consistently low, make sure there is not an underlying condition like anemia, hypothyroid, adrenal insufficiency, infection, Fibromyalgia, low blood sugar, depression or cancer. Blood tests and a physical exam can help rule out a medical problem. Also check any prescriptions or over the counter medications you are taking to see if fatigue might be a side effect.

I hope these ideas help you increase your energy. May your nights be restful and your days filled with liveliness and light.

Back Pain

In my practice the biggest complaint I hear from clients is, "My back hurts." When I ask them if they stretch they typically answer "No." or "Not enough." And most admit to sitting too much, either at their office or in the car. Here are some back care hints for you sitters.

Get up and move

It is essential to change position and tasks and move your body throughout the day. We are not made to sit in one posture for very long. It's recommended that you take a break at least every 50 minutes. This might be a quick walk around the block or your office or simply a three to five minute stretch. Do what feels good and don't push yourself to contort your body into positions that are painful. Basic moves like touching your toes, bending from side to side and stretching out your arms and neck are appropriate.

Chairs

You don't have to own the most expensive chair in the world, but you do have to make sure it fits YOUR body. We are all biologically individual and what feels good to me, might not feel good to you. If you have the option, pick out your own office chair after trying several options in the store. One that has adjustable arms, lumbar support and variable seat height is ideal. If you can't get a new chair, try to adapt the one you have with pillows or lumbar supports. The same applies to your car seat; take advantage of the built in adjustments available in your particular car and add additional pillows or lifts as needed to reach maximum comfort and support.

Stay active

If your job requires you to be seated a lot, pick leisure activities that get you moving. Passive activities like knitting, video games or checkers only encourage more sitting. Walk, jog, swim, hike or do yoga, whatever gets you up and moving. And if you do choose sedentary free-time activities, make sure you take breaks to move around and stretch.

No pain, no gain

What if even the shortest amount of sitting is a problem for you? It might be that you have a leg length difference. To some degree, we all have a shorter leg and it doesn't usually bother us. But some really feel it and it causes pain with prolonged standing or sitting. A chiropractor or massage therapist can usually tell you if your pelvis is tilted or legs are uneven. If this turns out to be true for you, using a lift in one shoe or a butt-lift when you are sitting can provide a huge relief. Chiropractors can often correct the leg length difference through treatment.

To determine which is your shorter leg, stand in bare feet and take a small book or magazine about ½ inch thick. Put it under one foot; stand evenly on both feet and see how you feel. Does it make you feel really crooked or even you out? Try it under the other foot. Inevitably, it feels good under one and horrible under the other. (Usually the short leg is the painful side of the back, but not always.) Now that you have determined your short side, use an insole in that one shoe or fold a pillow case and put it under that one side of your bottom when you are sitting. It can make all the difference in the world!

Get bodywork

Sometimes your back pain might be simply caused by muscle tension or a vertebra that has subluxed or gone out of alignment. A therapeutic massage can ease the muscle tension and a chiropractor can fix the subluxed vertebrae.

You may have been told that you have a herniated disc, ruptured disc, narrowing of the nerve passage or some other structural problem. I still encourage trying massage. Even though you could potentially have one of those serious structural issues, in some cases it is just the soft tissue that is causing the pain.

I always consider surgery a final resort after trying less invasive modalities. For example, I have had clients diagnosed with herniated discs who were on the verge of undergoing surgery. But after a few massages, the muscles loosened and the pain went away.

Stop needling me

Try acupuncture. More and more people are turning to acupuncture for low back pain. Jennifer Henry, LAC who suffered from back pain herself (www.theacupuncturelady.com) specializes in orthopedic acupuncture and has this to say about needling and back pain: "Acupuncture treats pain by increasing blood and energy flow in the effected tissues while also stimulating the release of endorphins and other pain killing neurotransmitters. It has been shown that over time, chronic pain makes changes in the brain's chemistry that reinforces the pain cycle. Acupuncture can reduce pain to a manageable level, reduce or eliminate the need for pain medications and increase the ability to cope with pain."

Mind/body connection

When we think of back pain, we assume that it is a physical problem: we sit too much, we lifted incorrectly, or we overdid that weekend soccer game. I have repeatedly observed a significant connection between the emotions and back pain. According to Louise Hay's *Heal Your Body A-Z*[48], back pain is associated with lack of emotional support, guilt, fear of money and financial support. I was taught that the low back corresponds with issues of sex, money and

---

[48] Hay, Louise. (1998). Heal Your Body A-Z. Hay House Inc.

personal relationship. Many clients that I see are having major problems in one or more of these areas.

We have a vast vocabulary that supports the idea that the mind and body are connected. For example, we might feel "unsupported", "stabbed in the back", that the "weight of the world is on our shoulders" or that we are "spineless" or "unstable". I believe that sometimes we have pain in our bodies to bring these emotions to the surface so they can be addressed. Or, pain erupts to draw our attention away from uncomfortable emotions like anger and depression. If you have back pain, explore issues of irritation and frustration. Acknowledge your emotions, talk them out and see if your pain starts to subside. Another good resource for exploring mind/body connection in relationship to pain is Dr. John Sarno's book, *Healing Back Pain*.[49]

I hope you never have to deal with back pain, but if you do, I hope these hints can help.

---

[49] Dr. John Sarno. (1991). Healing Back Pain. Warner Books.

Sleep

Early to bed and early to rise keeps a man healthy, wealthy and wise. Clearly Ben Franklin didn't have cats, children, deadlines, a spouse that snored, or a neighbor with a loud dog. Sleep is very important to maintain good health. It is during sleep that our bodies regenerate and heal, our minds rest and wander and through our dreams that our subconscious gets to play. Many ponder how much sleep we really need. There is no right answer to that question. As we grow and age we need different amounts of sleep and it is a myth that <u>everyone</u> needs eight hours. Some people function fine on six or seven, while others need nine or ten. We are all biologically individual and the most important thing is the quality of our sleep and that we sleep when we are tired. In today's stressful society, more and more people are developing sleep disorders and there are solutions other than prescription drugs. Here are some tips if you have problems; remember sleeplessness is not just an Ambien deficiency.

Daytime activities matter. Limit your caffeine intake and don't use stimulants to force yourself to stay awake, especially at night. We have a very delicate system of biorhythms and when you start to force yourself to stay awake later than you should, it alters your natural sleep cycle and you may start to experience sleep problems. Energy drinks like RedBull and RockStar only act as a temporary fix. Despite the boost of energy these drinks initially provide, you will eventually crash. They can also be highly addictive.

If you need a boost during the day try a walk, deep breathing, drinking water or having a healthy snack like nuts. Often when we hit that afternoon slump, we are dehydrated and just need more water or fresh air. Both transport oxygen in our system, which is needed for energy. Don't reach for sugary snacks, as they too can cause a crash. And avoid long naps, as that can result in evening wakefulness.

Another important component of good sleep is nutrition. Supplements like B vitamins, magnesium, tryptophan and melatonin may help you sleep. Make sure you don't take B vitamins too late in the day as they can cause wakefulness. Tryptophan is an essential amino acid, that our bodies cannot produce on their own and is one of the hardest to absorb from food sources, especially for vegetarians. Tryptophan, after a very unfair recall, is finally back on the market. It is the precursor to 5HTP which converts to Serotonin, the feel good hormone in the brain that helps with mood and sleep. Melatonin is another naturally occurring substance that can be taken as a supplement to help with sleep. However, avoid tryptophan or melatonin supplements if you are taking SSRI (Selective Serotonin Reuptake Inhibitor) drugs like Prozac and follow any dosing instructions on the label.

So, you have cut back on the caffeine, taken tryptophan and you STILL can't sleep. Let's talk about the sleep environment. Make sure the room is dark and quiet; use a white noise machine or earplugs if the space around you tends to be noisy, and make sure your pillows and mattress are appropriate for your unique body type.

Try not to do anything exciting before bed, like engaging in strenuous exercise or watching a loud scary movie. (Sex is ok.) Instead, choose activities that help you to relax and unwind from your day like reading a non-work related book, watching something fun on TV (not the news, which can frustrate us), petting your dog or cat, or taking a bubble bath or soak in the hot tub. It is time to leave the day behind us and rest. I know that can be difficult for those Type A executives and workaholics, but you have to distract yourself from the day how ever you can. And avoid excess alcohol at night. Not only is it a depressant, but it can disrupt sleep and cause dehydration.

Our minds seem to be our biggest obstacle to going to sleep. Often when we lay in bed, the dark and quiet gives our mind free reign to run rampant. We dwell on our day, worry about tomorrow, have fatalistic thoughts, wonder if what we did was wrong, question our choices for the future or simply lie there and do work in our heads. We ponder our to-do list or try to solve that one last problem. We have to find a way to shut off that thinker and relax. However, this is the toughest barrier to sleep because the mind can be like an unruly child. And there are times we really DO have work to do. What is the solution? As I see it, there are two options: shut up and sleep, or get up and work. I don't think it's bad to get out of bed and deal with things. To lie for hours thinking about something is pointless; get up and finish the paper, write stuff down, make a list for tomorrow, check to see if you actually made the deposit in the bank. These things are just going to drive you nuts if you don't address them, so go do them and then return to bed. Or just get up and distract yourself: read your book until you're tired, watch TV, do a Sudoku-anything to take your mind off the repeating thoughts. Meditation is another popular method for shutting off the mind. There are tapes available that you can play that lead you through a guided meditation to help relax your mind.

Or try to change your thought patterns. We can only think one thing at a time. So, if you are thinking about something negative or work related, change the thought to something else. This is what counting sheep is all about; it distracts the mind from other repetitive thoughts. Positive affirmations are another valuable tool to change thought patterns. If I find something is bothering me I will change the thought to "I fall asleep quickly and easily" or "I awake feeling refreshed." These affirmations not only distract you from the problem thoughts, but also program the body. Remember the mind/body connection and that we are the boss of them both.

Lastly, I would like to suggest some herbs and homeopathics. I recommend trying these before turning to the doctor for a prescription. Herbal teas containing hops, lavender, chamomile and valerian root are great for sleep.

There are also some wonderful homeopathic formulas like MoonDrops that allow you to drift off and not wake up feeling groggy. I encourage you to experiment and see what works best for you. Pleasant dreams!

Office Health in the Winter Season

When the cold and flu season is upon us, expect sneezes, sniffling and snot from the coworker who just borrowed your stapler. In an ideal world, people would not show up to work sick. But with the economy the way it is and people apprehensive about missing work for fear of losing a paycheck or losing their job, we must take the initiative to protect our own health. Here are some tips to keep you healthy in the workplace during winter.

Hygiene

Let's start with the basics. Our mothers were right; hand washing can protect you from germs. Make sure you wash your hands with soap and hot water and get between your fingers and under your fingernails. I know a lot of office staff that keep hand sanitizer at their desks and disinfectant wipes close by in case they are covering someone else's phone or using their supplies. In between hand washing, avoid touching your face and eyes too. Don't become too germ-phobic though, as being around germs can actually help you build up your immune system.

Supplements

Taking a multivitamin containing extra vitamin C and zinc has been shown to help prevent colds and speed recovery time. Some people mega dose on vitamin C, but we can only absorb a certain amount at a time (opinions vary on how much), so if you are going to take extra vitamin C, spread out the dose. Too much vitamin C can cause loose bowel movements and gas, which is a good hint that you've had too much. I personally am a big fan of Airborne. ™ Airborne was developed by a teacher and contains 17 vitamins, minerals and herbs. I find it works for me and could work well for you too.

Herbs like Echinacea and Golden Seal have properties that can help speed healing of colds and flu. Garlic is another helpful herb and can be taken in your food or bought in a "de-smelled" supplement form like Kyolic™. There are numerous supplement formulas on the market to boost your immune system; I recommend trying some and seeing what you like best.

Homeopathy

Homeopathics are a safe and easy way to try to stave off illness. Homeopathy works on the principle of "like cures like" and the remedy is determined by examining a combination of very specific symptoms like: Is your entire nose stuffy or just the right side? Does your headache get better when you drink cold water? Are you craving salt? Is your face flushed? Are you cranky and want to be left alone? Answering a series of questions such as these can guide you to the right single remedy.

Combination remedies are also readily available and tend to mingle the most common remedies for the ailment. There are remedies simply named Cold and Flu and there is an effective combination called Oscillococcinum™ which has worked for me in the past. You can inquire at your favorite health food store or contact a trained professional.

(For more info on homeopathy, see pg 14)

Think Yourself Well

We have enormous power in our mind. I fully believe that we can talk ourselves in and out of being sick. If you are afraid of every germ and sure that so and so from your office is infecting you, chances are you are going to catch something. Our attitude and what we say in our minds strongly effects what happens in our bodies. Repeating to yourself that you are healthy and well or that your immune system is strong can actually prevent you from catching the latest thing.

De-stress Yourself!

So much research has been done on the effects of stress on the immune system. And let's be clear, it is not so much the stress, it's your <u>reaction</u> to the stress. If you can take things in stride and make sure you are allowing yourself some downtime to process all of what is happening in your life, you can keep that immune system healthier.

Keep Drinking Water

Not only should we have a large amount of water for health in general, but it is even more important when we are sick. Water can help thin out mucous and keep our noses and lungs clear. Tea, broth and juice are good too, just make sure you are not adding artificial sweeteners or getting juice that is filled with high-fructose corn syrup.

Try to be as Happy as you Can

I have studied people who are always sick. You know them; they catch everything that comes around. And they always try to blame someone for "getting them sick". I have noticed that more often than not, these people are basically unhappy. Perhaps they don't like their jobs; maybe their marriage is less than ideal, or they could be experiencing some level of depression. Whatever the source of the unhappiness, I think that if they can be happier, they will also be healthier. Illness is very often used as an excuse to not face something. I would suggest to someone that is always sick that they examine what else is going on in their lives. It is sometimes a really hard question to ask ourselves, but worth the work if we desire to stay healthy and have a long and productive life.

Western Medicine

What about Western Medicine? What does it have to offer at this time of year? Not much frankly. Right now people are rushing to get their flu shots. These are recommended for older adults, children and people with compromised immune systems. Every year the formula changes in an effort to battle the virus of the year. Some people have found the flu shot makes them sick, and others get the flu anyway. I have read numerous reports that the flu shot increases the risk for Alzheimer's disease from the additives like mercury and aluminum contained in the vaccine.[50]

I have also seen evidence that the vaccine doesn't do anything at all.[51] Remember that the flu shot is a combination of many chemical and natural compounds, some of which can have side effects. I am not recommending against the flu shot, but rather encouraging you to be informed before you make any medical or natural health choice.

Antibiotics are not going to help you get rid of a cold either. A cold is caused by a virus and antibiotics work on bacteria. However, if a cold develops into an upper respiratory infection or sinus infection, antibiotics may be appropriate. Some doctors recommend flu anti-virals which are effective if taken at the first signs of being sick (within the first two days). It can decrease the length of the flu by one or two days and makes you less contagious to others according to the CDC website. These specific drugs will not work on a cold, just the flu.

And remember, the sneezing, runny nose, coughing that comes with a cold is the body's effort to get the bad stuff out. If you go overboard in repressing the symptoms with drugs, you may prolong the illness. One of your best defenses is rest, so try to get plenty of it and take the time off work if possible!

---

[50] http://www.wellnessresources.com/health/articles/are_vaccinations_causing_early_onset_alzheimers_disease/ (This is just one example, many are out there.)

[51] http://www.tanplusforhealth.com/news/november/flu_shot.htm

I hope you all make it through this winter season healthy, well and disease free. But if you do happen to catch something, I hope these natural health hints make it an easier time for you. Good luck and good health!

Natural Solutions for Depression
and Anxiety

More people than ever are experiencing depression and other mood disorders. These are commonly treated with antidepressants. In the pharmaceutical world, antidepressants rank number five in numbers of prescriptions written behind those for high blood pressure, cholesterol, gastrointestinal disorders and antibiotics.

Although it is recommended to treat serious, debilitating depression with antidepressants and psychotherapy, there are non-drug ways to treat mild depression and its mental sister, anxiety.

The first thing I look at with my clients is nutrition. Many people suffering from depression and anxiety are low in B vitamins and I suggest adding a daily B supplement. Be aware not to take them too late in the day as they can disrupt sleep. Tryptophan and 5HTP are precursors to serotonin which controls mood and are great additions to your daily regimen. SAM-e, Melatonin, Omega 3 fatty acids and St. Johns Wort are also beneficial supplement suggestions if you are battling mood disorders. But it is not recommended to take St John's Wort, Tryptophan or 5-HTP if you are on SSRIs (Selective Serotonin Reuptake Inhibitors) like Prozac, as there can be a dangerous interaction.[52]

If you are experiencing anxiety, cut back on the caffeine and other stimulants. Even if you have been drinking it for years, with the addition of stressful life circumstances, caffeine can increase your feelings of anxiety. Taper off slowly so the withdrawal symptoms don't send you back to the java. Also avoid self-medicating with alcohol. It,

---

[52] Gaby, Alan & Healthnotes Medical Team, Inc. (Eds.) (2006) A-Z Guide to Drug-Herb-Vitamin Interactions. (2nd ed.).

in itself, is a depressant and can just lead down a road to addiction and isolation.

I also suggest eliminating artificial sweeteners and flavorings like MSG. I have had clients that have experienced anxiety-like symptoms after consuming artificial sweeteners. As soon as they eliminated the artificial sweeteners from their diets, the symptoms went away. Keeping a food diary is a great way to pinpoint food sensitivities and can also be useful to chart correlations between eating and mood changes. You can also be tested for heavy metal contamination, which can affect both mood and food allergies. And it never hurts to do a cleanse or short fast. The cleaner the colon, the better off we are.

A lot of people are on multiple prescription drugs and I advise checking side effects to make sure they are not experiencing iatrogenic disease. (Loosely meaning 'treatment induced'). Many antidepressants have anxiety as a side effect and vice versa. Also, studies have shown that low cholesterol aggravates depression, so make sure your statin drug is not lowering your numbers too much.[53]

SAD or Seasonal Affective Disorder is common during the winter months. Using a light box or supplementing with vitamin D can help with this issue. Make sure you get out in the light for the time that we have it. While you are outside, exercise a bit. Dr. Andrew Weil suggests that 30 minutes a day, five days a week can help with mood issues. Exercise not only gets you outside and around other people, but it boosts your self-confidence by releasing those feel good hormones in the brain.

We cannot escape the connection of body and mind and studies have shown that massage and acupuncture can help the symptoms of depression and anxiety. Massage, in general, relaxes the body and also stimulates the brain's feel good hormones. The state of relaxation can also alleviate

---

[53] http://www.priory.com/psych/cholesterol.htm (This website quotes numerous useful studies about not only depression but increased risk of violence and suicide with lowered cholesterol.)

mild anxiety. A study conducted in 2000 by John Allen at the University of Tucson, showed that over 50% of people treated with acupuncture for their depression had lessening of symptoms to a level so that they no longer met the criteria for depression.

Other alternatives to prescription drugs are homeopathics or Bach Flower Essences. Both work on the premise that "like cures like" and work on an energetic level. They balance the body so that healing can take place from within. Flower essences correspond to specific emotional states and restore them to balance. There are millions of combinations that are individualized for every person. More information on Bach Flower Essences can be found at www.bachflower.com. A great website to help you narrow down a homeopathic formula is www.abchomeopathy.com and please see page 33 for in depth information about Bach Flower Essences.

Just as two solid objects cannot occupy the same space at one time, you cannot hold two thoughts in your mind at one time. If you are having negative thoughts, replace them with positive ones. Affirmations, or positive statements of transformation, are an excellent means of changing your thought patterns. For example, rather than saying, "Life sucks," change it to "Life is abundant and easy." Instead of saying "I am getting sick," say "I am healthy and well." When working with affirmations make them short, positive and in the present. And repeat frequently. I have affirmations around the house on my mirrors and on the dash board of my car. It is a helpful reminder that we are in control of the stories we tell and the visions we create for our life path. Affirmations can help shape your reality rather than feeling like a victim to your own life.

If you are experiencing depression or anxiety, try talking to a professional about it. No matter what treatment you are using, it is important to cover the cognitive aspect of depression and anxiety as well. And remember, you don't have to go through this alone. Bonding with people and companion animals is important. When in this state it is also advised to skip horror movies, news programs and other shows that add anxiety and reinforce a negative state of mind.

Be Your Own Advocate

We assume that when we go to a hospital or are under a doctor's care that we are in a safe and trustworthy environment. My experience, especially lately has been that you have to check and double-check the care that you are getting. Incorrect prescriptions have been given to the wrong patients, food might not be delivered and on the extreme end of the spectrum, wrong limbs have been removed. Hospitals are understaffed, nurses are overworked and doctors have become a prescription pad. What can you do to make certain that you are getting the best care?

~ Ask questions

Medical professionals have a habit of tossing a bunch of Latin at you; hoping parts of it are understood. I have also observed them imparting detailed and complicated information to partially unconscious patients in a hospital bed. During meetings, many patients nod their head and only later realize they don't understand the information received. Don't be embarrassed if you don't immediately comprehend something a doctor or nurse tells you. There are no stupid questions when it comes to your health. Ask them to clarify.

Great questions to keep in mind are: "How long will this last?", "Are there any side effects with that drug?", "What will that test show?", "Can you explain what those results mean?"

And make sure you get copies of your blood work and test results and file them. You have a right to see your own test results and it can clear up questions later if you develop a condition and need to check for patterns, or switch medical professionals. I believe you cannot have too much information about your condition, medication or projected outcome.

Some people get very nervous or self conscious when they see their doctor and often forget to ask questions. This is understandable, especially if you have a serious condition. Prepare your questions in advance in writing when you are calm and have time to think. Talk to others who may have had the same diagnosis or symptoms; often they will know things that you would never think to ask. Capitalize on their expertise and input.

~ <u>Do your own research</u>

So, you have received a Latin name or set of initials for your condition (IBS, PMS, RLS, ALS, PTSD, it goes on ad infinitum...that's Latin). Well, what the heck does it mean? A great way to be your own advocate is to develop some medical knowledge by doing your own research on your condition. Information is power, and the more you understand, the easier it will be to communicate with your doctor and ask informed questions.

When your physician explains a diagnosis, it is very important to understand everything you have just been told. Doctors often have handouts or will give you as much time as you need to have it explained to you. A lot have limited time however, so you might walk out of the office with a few initials and a prescription. This is where YOUR research comes in. With the advent of the internet we can find information about anything. This is both good and bad. I have had clients thoroughly convinced that they were dying because of something they read on the internet. I know others who have researched their condition so thoroughly, that they could teach their doctors a thing or two.

Common ailments are easy to locate on line and many have support groups or bulletin boards where you can post questions and comments. One concern about the internet is that it gives everyone a voice or platform to share their opinion or self-appointed expertise, regardless of credentials or motive. Thus be careful where you get your information. Don't believe every post on every bulletin board and don't rely too heavily on blogs and notes from laypeople. Web MD is a reliable source for medical information as are most sites affiliated with a university or hospital. Also, double check your information by using multiple sites.

Now, what if you prefer to take a more alternative approach to your disease, dysfunction or disorder? There are great resources for that as well. Again, check to see who is sponsoring each site you visit and don't rely on just ONE for your information. www.theholisticoption.com is a great place to start and sites associated with large foundations are also pretty reputable. Be ware of sites that have information posted just to sell you their newest product. The information might be valid, but could also be a propaganda sales pitch. Remember, you can find information to support any theory on the internet so be discerning.

~ Seek out more

Don't be afraid to get a second, third, or fourth opinion if something doesn't sound or feel right to you. Not every medical professional knows everything. Commonly, things are misdiagnosed or over/under diagnosed. You might have to convince your insurance company to cover further tests or diagnoses, but do it if you feel it is needed.
Unfortunately, most insurance companies are more concerned about making money, than advocating for your wellness, so fight for what you need.

~ Know thyself

It is so important for us to be in touch with our bodies and to know if something feels right or not. Trust yourself. You are living inside your body and know it better than anyone else. Know how you react to certain medications, how your muscles and bones feel and your energy level and sleep patterns. Also track how medication makes you feel.

I had a client who was taking a very potent seizure medication for her headaches. She came to my office with symptoms I suspected were side effects from this drug. The more she took the drug, the worse the side effect symptoms became. Her doctor wanted to give her ADDITIONAL drugs for these new conditions. (This phenomenon of prescriptions causing new symptoms is called iatrogenic disease.) I finally asked her if the headache medicine was even working and she confessed that after six months her headaches hadn't changed at all. She was afraid to tell her doctor, but I encouraged her to. He pulled her off the medications and though her headaches were still there, all the other problems disappeared. Sometimes you have to be your own detective. Owning a *PDR, (Prescription Drug Reference)*, is a big help. You can also find common side effects on-line. And sometimes the side effects can be worse than the initial condition.

~ Get help

Imagine the following scenario: you have been admitted to the hospital while your family is far away and you are too sick to do your own research. Instead of accepting this situation, find someone to act as your advocate. This can be as simple as friends who can double check information or a paid caregiver. It is particularly important to have someone there when a doctor is explaining things to you: especially if you are sick, weak, exhausted or unconscious. It is also useful to have someone present to make sure you are eating, wearing your hearing aid or glasses, double-checking what medications you are receiving, taking you to the bathroom, etc. If you have no one to help, there are volunteer advocates and people that are paid for this service. Some hospitals even provide them. Search on-line for an advocate service in your area or ask at the facility where you are staying.

A client of mine was recently in the hospital and without anyone asking if it was needed, a stool softener was prescribed. This patient had previously had his gall bladder removed and was thus already prone to loose stool. Due to this oversight, this patient found himself trying to rush to the bathroom attached to an IV, releasing his bowels all over himself, the bed, the floor and his booties. The nurse was informed to take the stool softener off the chart. Later that day, another stool softener arrived with the pills. Luckily we caught it before it was given. Two more stool softeners arrived over the next two days because no one ever took it off the chart. These things happen and it can be a lot more serious than just poo!

Although we want to believe in the infallibility of our medical professionals, the reality is that no one is perfect and everyone can make a mistake. Take control, ask questions and be your own best advocate!

A side note: There are fabulous physicians, hospitals and nurses. I am by no means implying that everyone is incompetent, but in the case of your health, it is better to be safe than sorry.

Cancer

There are certain phrases that people dread hearing in their lifetime, "Let's just be friends", "We have to talk", and "You have cancer". The last can instill fear and panic in the hearts of even the strongest people. Since the war on cancer began things have only gotten worse and you may wonder if modern medicine has the weapons needed to fight the war properly. Perhaps the mêlée should be fought on a smaller battlefield, inside each of us. What can we do to protect ourselves from cancer and fight it off if diagnosed with it?

Cancer is the uncontrolled replication of cells. This happens all the time in our bodies and the immune system deals with the problem. When cancer takes hold however, we must boost the immune system to help fight. But what are some things that lead to cancer?

Studies have linked a high fat diet to increased risk of breast and colon cancer.[54] Cutting back on foods that are heavy in saturated fats like red meat and processed foods can help reduce that risk. Increasing foods that are rich in phytochemicals such as fruits and vegetables help keep your immune system strong and eliminate free-radicals. Also, estrogen has been shown to be related to breast and uterine cancer, among others.[55],[56]. Estrogen is stored in body fat, so maintaining a healthy weight is valuable.

We all know that smoking is bad news leading to both lung and bladder cancers, and that we should avoid this nasty habit. Luckily, in California, legislation was passed

---

[54] A diet high in fat significantly increases a woman's risk of developing invasive breast cancer, according to a study conducted by researchers at the National Cancer Institute in Bethesda, Maryland, and published in the Journal of the National Cancer Institute.

[55] http://www.breastcancer.org/treatment/hormonal/what_is_it/hormone_role.jsp

[56] http://www.cumc.columbia.edu/news/in-vivo/Vol2_Iss10_may26_03/index.html

that prohibits smoking in bars and restaurants and makes it illegal to smoke within 20 feet of the entrance to a public building. Many other states have followed suit. Although this 20 foot law is helpful, smoke follows its own rules and inevitably seems to flow toward the nearest non-smoker. Avoid being in enclosed areas such as cars while someone is smoking and definitely avoid smoking around children and pets.

The second leading cause of lung cancer, after smoking, is exposure to radon gas. Radon comes up through the ground from rock, specifically uranium. According to the National Cancer Institute, Radon contributes to 15,000 to 22,000 lung cancer deaths per year[57]. Testing is the only way to know if your home has radon leakage. The largest amount accumulates in the basement or first floor and tends to be in airtight homes. Radon can also come from well water and building materials. Tests can be obtained by calling 1-800-SOS-RADON.

Another danger of being in tightly sealed homes is the out gassing from carpet, furniture and paint. California leads the nation in the strictest paint and chemical regulations and has passed a no VOC (Volatile Organic Compounds) law. There are low or non VOC options, but they tend to be more pricey; costing 15-20 % more than the conventional products. Though some indoor air pollution is known to be cancer causing in animals and some humans, most are not considered a direct cause of cancer. However, some people develop sensitivity to out gassed chemicals and overtime a build up or combination of them can lead to health issues. If you are using products such as paint, solvents, glues, or air fresheners, it is recommended by the EPA[58] that you increase ventilation, dispose of the containers properly and avoid allowing children and pets to inhale the fumes.

---

[57] Cancer and Radon. Retrieved Feb. 23, 2008 from www.cancer.gov

[58] http://www.epa.gov/iaq/voc.html

Pesticides and herbicides that are sprayed on agricultural land and in parks are a contributing factor to disease. *The Organic Resource Guide* published by The Pesticide Awareness and Alternative Coalition, estimates that there are over 400 chemicals regularly used in conventional farming in Santa Barbara County.[59] The coalition recommends, as do most anti-cancer organizations, eating organic foods that are not genetically modified or sprayed with chemicals.

Though we have seen a large increase in the availability and consumption of organic products, we are still inundated with "Franken-foods." These are foods that have been genetically modified or altered, which are also called GMOs or Genetically Modified Organisms. Right now some of our largest crops are GMO; corn and soy being the most prevalent. Monsanto, a multi-national company is leading the way in patenting GM seeds and genetically modifying our foods. They are making billions and we are being subjected to, what I believe to be, the biggest human science experiment in history. Regulations are very lax in this country regarding these practices and the food is not only assumed to be safe without much testing, but labeling is not a requirement. Beware of foods containing high fructose corn syrup and soybean oil since these not only indicate a highly processed food, but also one that is probably genetically modified.

You may be wondering what genetically modified foods have to do with cancer. Well, unfortunately the jury is still out on that subject. Since these foods were not thoroughly tested before release and we don't know ultimately how these modifications are going to affect our own DNA, or combine with each other we cannot predict what the ramifications will be. I advise you to avoid GMOs and let your grocers and government know you won't tolerate these current food practices.

---

[59] The Organic Resource Guide published by The Pesticide Awareness and Alternative Coalition. Page 7.

Californians are lucky to have such a large amount of local, organic farms. However, large scale farms that use conventional growing practices still use poisonous sprays and chemicals that not only affect our food, but contaminate our ground water and coastal water. Even if we are not eating this food directly, much of it is used in feed for animals that we will end up eating. In 2004, Santa Barbara County ranked 12th in the state for pesticide use and it was estimated that 4,109,252 pounds were used, mainly on strawberries and grapes for wine production.[60]

With every bar code that is scanned, we send an important message about what we want as consumers. Frequenting farmers markets and local stands and choosing organic produce over conventionally grown produce can send the message to the government that safe food is important to us. Recently, the local public's voice was heard when the City of Santa Barbara voted that 19 of our 56 parks would be pesticide-free with the rest to follow suit. Since the EPA revealed that children receive 50% of their lifetime cancer risk in the first two years of life, this is an important move for the health of our children.[61] To change laws like this in your area, contact the mayor or city council.

Besides eating organic food and cutting back on saturated fats, what else can we do to stay healthy? How about exercise? Exercise reduces body fat, boosts immune function and gives you a good outlook on life. According to Sara Rosenthal, author of *Stopping Cancer at the Source*, "Exercise stimulates the production of endorphins; neurotransmitters that occur naturally in the brain and make us feel good. It brings oxygen to our blood and the more oxygen in the blood, the less hospitable the environment to cancer." [62]

---

[60] Central Coast Environmental health Project, ccehp.org.

[61] The Organic Resource Guide published by The Pesticide Awareness and Alternative Coalition. Page 1.

[62] Rosenthal, M.S. (2001). Stopping Cancer at the Source. Canada: Trafford Publishing. Pg. 72-73.

Where you exercise is also important. I have observed countless people running and cycling on very busy streets. Not only does this increase your risk of getting hit by a car, but you are breathing noxious fumes from automobiles and busses. Ground level ozone from car exhaust, brake dust and tire burn off has been shown to contribute to lung disease and respiratory problems.[63] Even with some of the strictest auto emissions standards in the country, we still have an enormous number of cars spewing chemicals into our air. We have many bike paths, beaches and mountain trails; try your exercise in a more natural environment.

What if we do find ourselves with a cancer diagnosis? Though chemotherapy, radiation and surgery are offered by Western medicine, there are far less invasive natural alternatives that can boost your healing.

Increase vitamin C. I mean tons of it. Bowel tolerance is a way to tell when the body is done accepting it. If you spread the doses throughout the day, it's more easily tolerated and absorbed. Too much causes diarrhea, so you don't want to get to that point. If it happens, back off the dose.

It's believed that cancer cannot live in an oxygen-rich or alkalized environment. Deep breathing is beneficial as is a hyperbaric chamber if you can find one. A hyperbaric chamber looks like a tanning bed and delivers oxygen at a pressure higher than atmospheric. The patient stays in for 30-90 minutes and this high pressure oxygen can help cellular health, anti-aging and clearing toxic residue[64]. Liquid Oxygen is available from health food stores to drip into water. As far as alkalinity goes, there are supplements available in most health food stores, as well as filtration systems that alkalize the drinking water. Also, a diet rich in

---

[63] Rosenthal, M.S. (2001) Stopping Cancer at the Source. Canada: Trafford Publishing. Pg. 201.

[64] http://www.hyperbaricchambertreatment.com/

green leafy vegetables and other alkaline foods can contribute to a state of alkalinity

Studies have shown how important attitude is with cancer outcome. A fighting spirit wins. This is the biggest competition you will ever be in and fighting and staying positive will work wonders. Surround yourself with people who love you and tell them to remain positive when around you. Prayer is very powerful and people in a group thinking the same healing thoughts can be very beneficial.

Eliminating anything processed is recommended. Chemicals and preservatives in food just give your body something else to fight. Whole foods, fruits and vegetables are key. I personally recommend avoiding wheat and dairy as they can be hard on the digestive system. Keeping up nutrition is very important and a good multivitamin, mineral and amino acid formula would be valuable. Some experts recommend a macrobiotic diet, or at the very least going organic and vegetarian. If you can handle the restrictions, these dietary changes can be beneficial, but make sure you get enough protein and amino acids.

It's not only important to be selective about what we are putting IN our bodies, but also ON our bodies. One of the most commonly used products is deodorant containing aluminum. We are smearing this daily on some of the most absorbent tissue in the body. Though no specific link is found between deodorant and cancer, I would avoid this, especially if you have already had a breast cancer diagnosis.[65] Also avoid creams, lotions, cosmetics and sunscreens that contain non-organic products.

I HIGHLY recommend testing for both heavy metals and environmental toxin exposure, depending on where you grew up, where you live now and any potential exposure pertinent to your occupation. Both tests are simple; the presence of metal contaminants in the body can be determined by testing a hair sample and environmental toxins can be determined by a simple blood test. You can

[65] http://www.cancer.gov/cancertopics/factsheet/Risk/AP-Deo

consult a natural medicine doctor or naturopath to order those tests. If the results come back positive, it would be beneficial to do a cleanse or chelation therapy to flush the chemicals out.

The following suggestions are from numerous sources:

There is a product called Wo-Benzymes that has shown great effect of decreasing tumor size and boosting the immune system.[66]

In a recent article on Soothing the Pain of Chemotherapy. The article recommended 1000mg Green Tea Extract, 20mg melatonin (at bedtime for sleep) and a multivitamin with at least 1000mg of vitamin C. Another source recommends melatonin at night saying it increased survival and improved quality of life.

Zinc is a great supplement for boosting the immune system and 150mg/day can also help reduce the effects of radiation therapy.

N-Acetylcysteine (NAC) decreased the negative effects of chemotherapy agents. 1000mg, given 90 minutes before chemo treatment is recommended. [67]

There have been numerous doctors persecuted and forced out of the United States for their work on curing cancer. One is Dr. Hoxsey whose clinic is still functioning in Mexico and the other is a nurse named Rene Caisse.[68] She created a formula called Essiac which is still available at www.essiac-canada.com. I had a client that used this formula on her husband with melanoma and his recovery was much quicker than expected.

---

[66] http://www.breastcancerchoices.org/enzymes.html

[67] http://www.lifecheck.co.za/index2.php/?page_id=157

[68] http://essiacinfo.org

From the book *Prescription for Nutritional Healing*[69]:
Nutrients that are recommended:

Coenzyme Q10
Garlic
Melatonin
Omega 3 fatty acids (fish oil)
Wobenzymes
Shark Cartilage
Superoxide Dismutase (This can be injected by a doctor)
Vitamins A and E, B and C
Maitake, reishi and shiitake mushrooms are recommended to
boost the immune system and are considered to have
anti-tumor properties.
Acidophilus was suggested to help promote good bacteria in
the colon.
Grape seed extract is a powerful antioxidant and can help
boost the immune system.

The book *Prescription for Herbal Healing*[70] suggests
drinking licorice tea to help with nausea during
chemotherapy.

Reiki, which is a hands-on healing technique can help
with attitude, energy and possibly help decrease the cancer.
You can look in the phone book or on-line for a practitioner
near you. I personally would find someone who has
practiced for more than five years and is master level.
Someone of the master level can teach you or your family to
do Reiki at home. See page 18 for more information on
Reiki.
Cancer and health are also affected by personal
attitude and mental outlook. As I have mentioned in previous
articles, I see a large correlation between what we think and

---

[69] Balch, Phyllis. Prescription for Nutritional Healing. 1997
[70] Balch, Phyllis. Prescription for Herbal Healing. 2002

what happens in our bodies. I believe one of the reasons we get sick is to let us know something is out of balance with our emotional/spiritual side. Our emotions need to let us know that something must change. When we ignore the emotions we open up the window for sickness. I also believe that malfunctions in our body are the body's way to communicate that something is wrong in our mind and spirit. I believe that if we don't acknowledge our emotional needs and issues, this energy has to go somewhere and manifests as illness or <u>dis-ease</u>. A child will only scream mommy, mommy, mommy, mommy for so long before he starts pulling things off shelves. This is also what our emotions do. The carpal tunnel, sciatica, neck pain, headaches, psoriasis and cancer is our emotional child pulling things off shelves because it has been ignored. I'm not saying that illness is 100% emotionally formed. There are toxins, poisons and hereditary components to consider. But if our emotions are even responsible for 10% of our illnesses and we can control them, why wouldn't we?

Visualization for healing cancer

Get into a relaxed place, in a comfortable position. Breathe deeply and try to quiet the mind. Get a picture in your head of what you think the cancer looks like. It can be a ball, a blob, whatever it is to you. Picture it in the area of the body where it is growing. As you inhale, send the breath to that organ and tumor and picture it shooting at it, eating it, dissolving it, whatever scene works for you. I always saw it as the cavalry coming over the hill in the old movies to save the day. That cavalry are your white blood cells and they are surrounding the tumor to get rid of it. Hold the picture of the tumor disappearing for as long as you can. Do this visualization as many times during the day as possible. I have seen amazing results with this type of meditation.

If you have already started chemotherapy, greet it as a positive thing. As it's going into your body, picture it fighting the cancer and see the tumors shrinking. If you fight against the chemo and dread it, or see it as a poisonous enemy, it will not work as well for you.

And last but not least, I encourage you to communicate with your health providers. Ask questions, do your own research and get a second, third and fourth opinion if necessary. And, if it is in your nature, seek out more natural cures such those we have covered above. We need to be our own advocate. Good luck and good health.

Natural Solutions for Acid Indigestion

Symptoms:

If you were diagnosed with acid indigestion (sour stomach or upset stomach) by your doctor, you may be experiencing any of the following symptoms:

- Abdominal Fullness
- Belching
- Heartburn, which is a sensation of warmth or burning located in the chest.

According to http://www.alkaseltzer.com/as/facts.htm [71] the burning & pressure of heartburn can last as long as two hours and is often provoked by bending over, lying down or eating certain foods. Occasional acid indigestion symptoms or heartburn is common in most people. However, frequent and severe acid indigestion or symptoms of heartburn may be signs of a serious condition that requires treatment.

Causes:

There are several possible causes of acid indigestion that can be addressed without pharmaceutical intervention. According to http://heartburn.about.com/cs/causes/a/ heartburncauses.htm [72], these are the most common foods that can cause indigestion:
- Coffee, tea and other caffeinated beverages
- Chocolate, which contains theobromine, a compound which relaxes the lower esophageal sphincter (LES) and can allow acid to squirt into the esophagus

---

[71] Acid Indigestion and Heartburn Facts. Retrieved March 6, 2007 from website: http://www.alkaseltzer.com/as/facts.htm

[72] 10 Most Frequent Causes of Heartburn. Retrieved March 6, 2007 from website: http://heartburn.about.com/cs/causes/a/ heartburncauses.htm

- Fried and fatty foods which tend to slow digestion
- Tomatoes and tomato-based products which can relax the LES
- Alcohol, which relaxes the LES and increases stomach acid
- Tobacco
- Citrus fruits and juices

Other contributing factors may be:
- Tight fitting clothing such as belts and slenderizing undergarments
- Eating too close to bedtime; lying down puts pressure on the LES, increasing the chance of refluxed food
- Eating large meals

Tenney in her book *Today's Herbal Health* says the following also contributes to indigestion:
- Eating too fast
- Poor food combinations
- Excess water with meals, which can dilute the stomach acid causing over production of acid to compensate
- Excessive use of raw foods
- Overeating

Dietary Changes:

Today's Herbal Health (Tenney, 1998) recommends a diet that will aid digestion and improve health. The diet suggests that whole grains (considered "primary foods") comprise 20-30% of your diet; protein by way of animal protein, tofu, tempeh and beans comprise another 20-30% of your diet; fresh, seasonal vegetables (contain "secondary foods") comprise 30-40% of your diet, and lastly, 5-10% of your diet should consist of fruits, eggs, dairy and oils

An elimination diet is another dietary method that can prove helpful in determining what is causing digestive and allergy problems. Typically an elimination diet entails eliminating wheat, dairy, soy, eggs, and corn for six weeks and slowly reintroducing the foods one by one, noting any changes along the way. Avoiding these common trigger foods to see if changes occur in the indigestion can also be very helpful. Keeping a food diary is another way to help identify problem foods and patterns.

A balanced diet that includes good amounts of first-class high protein foods such as meat, eggs and dairy is key to health. These foods help repair damage to tissues and cells and stimulate and maintain body metabolism. (Tierra, 1998) Healthy fats are also important in your diet. Trans fats (formed from hydrogenated and partially hydrogenated oils) should be avoided but the good fats like omega 3 and 6 found in nuts, avocados and olive oil are essential for healthy hair and skin and help with digestion of food. Healthy fats also contain necessary vitamins such as A, D, K and E. (Tierra, 1998)

There are different schools of thought on vitamin supplements. Some experts believe that if we consume enough of the right foods we don't need to supplement. Others say that it is impossible to get all the nutrients we need just though our food. There are herbal tonics and nutritive herbs available that can help complement your diet. You could also try a vitamin supplement. Once taking vitamins on a regular basis, some people feel healthier or that their immune systems are stronger. Gauge how you feel. Your body will let you know what you need.

Helpful Herbs and Spices for Digestive Health

There are several kitchen herbs that can be added to your meals to help thwart acid indigestion. These are commonly found herbs that you may already be using in your food preparation. A few suggestions are (Tierra 1998):
    - Drink a tea of basil leaves.
    - Add bay leaves to soups and stews.
    - Fennel is great for reducing gas and calming cramps.

- Ginger is one of the best digestive aids. Many countries serve crystallized ginger for dessert or in between courses to act as a carminative (digestive aid) and help digestion.
- Rosemary, a popular herb, can be used for indigestion, gas and nausea.

Richard Mabey in his book The New Age Herbalist (1988) recommends an infusion (strong tea) of fennel, mint, dill, chamomile, anise or lemon balm be taken after the meal to aid digestion.

Additional Herbal Remedies:

- **Hops** can be useful for both digestion and gas, and can help bring about relaxation. I prefer a tincture of hops which is made by distilling the herb in alcohol. I use a few drops in a glass of water as symptoms dictate.
- **Chamomile** is another helpful herb for digestion and relaxation. Commercially made chamomile tea is widely available and a cup of the tea following dinner and before bedtime has been shown to have beneficial properties.
- A tea of **slippery elm bark** can be taken to calm the burning pain of indigestion.
- **Marshmallow Root** (not to be confused with candy marshmallows) can be taken in capsules (2 before meals) or tea to soothe your stomach.
- A tablespoon of **bee pollen** before meals can aid digestion and also provides B, A, C, D and E vitamins. (Tenney, 1992) As a side note, local bee pollen can help with environmental allergies like hay fever. However, do not consume bee pollen if you are allergic to bee stings.
- Both **fennel** and **catnip** tea are helpful to children with colic and indigestion. A weak tea given several times a day as tolerated is recommended. (Tenney, 1992)
- A bitter herb like **Angelica** is often found in pre-dinner aperitifs to stimulate the appetite and enhance

digestion. It also helps the body absorb nutrients from the meal.

You can make your own cocktail with the following recipe:[73], [74]

> 1 ounce dried gentian root, ground and sifted
> ½ ounce dried barberry, ground and sifted
> ½ ounce dried angelica, ground and sifted
> ¼ ounce crushed dried fennel seeds
> ¼ ounce crushed dried cardamom seeds

Combine the ingredients, put them in a glass container with a tight-fitting lid, and store in a cool location (a kitchen cupboard will do fine). Then, to make a day's worth of apéritif, add 1 teaspoon of the herb mix to 1 cup of boiling water. Cover, and simmer for 15 minutes. Allow the drink to cool, then strain the herbs from the liquid. Have half a cup before lunch and the rest before dinner. It makes enough for 20 cups.

Remember that everyone is a unique individual and not all remedies work for every person. Experiment to see what works for you or talk to a professional.

Other suggestions

It is not only true that we are what we eat. We also "are what we think". Often times our bodies manifest our thoughts and emotions through physical illness. If you are suffering from acid indigestion you might want to ask yourself the following questions:

Is something eating at you?

Are emotions like anger or resentment bubbling up to the surface?

---

[73] A Five Herb Aperitif for Indigestion. Retrieved March 10, 2007 from website: http://www.prevention.com/article/0,5778,s1-1-52-112-3766-1,00.html

[74] Most cities around the country now have health food stores or bulk herb stores where you can purchase these products. If you don't have one near you, you can find mail order suppliers on-line.

Is something burning you up?

Frequently, through changing our minds, we can change our bodies.

Taking digestive enzymes with food can help support the digestive system and sometimes an occasional cleansing fast will allow your body's systems to rest. After the fast, slowly add in healthy, easily digested foods.

Another cause of indigestion is a deficiency of acid in the stomach. This condition is known as hypochlorhydria which can occur as we age. Low stomach acid can cause food to stagnate and putrefy in the stomach, which is later burped up. Acid is also required to trigger the LES to open and allow food to pass into the small intestine. If there is not enough acid, the sphincter will not open to allow the food to move out. You level of stomach acid can be checked with a Heidelberg test or by adding HCl (hydrochloric acid) and seeing how the body reacts. Do this under the guidance of a physician.

Book References

Mabey, Richard (1988) *The New Age Herbalist*, New York: Simon and Schuster.

Tenney, Louise MH (1992) *Today's Herbal Health*, Provo, UT: Woodland Publishing.

Tierra, Michael L.Ac, OMD (1998) *The Way of Herbs*, New York: Pocket Books.

Herbal Formula for High Blood Pressure

I have created an herbal combination for balancing high blood pressure. This is a common problem amongst my clients and if you suffer from hypertension, I believe this is a good product to have on hand. Furthermore, I encourage people to make it on their own. I have chosen a capsule form, as it has longer storage life than infusions and decoctions and therefore does not need to be made as frequently. In addition, I think our culture has adapted to taking pills, whether it is vitamins or pharmaceuticals, so the capsule method may more easily fit within an already established routine.

Herbs included in this formula: 1 part Garlic, 1 part Hawthorn, ½ part Ginkgo Biloba, ½ part Valerian Root, ¼ part Peppermint Leaf (optional).

Garlic [75], which helps to expand vessel walls, lowers serum cholesterol, provides rapid and prolonged decrease in blood pressure, inhibits the tendency of blood cells to stick together and reduces the tendency of blood to clot in both animal and human studies.

Hawthorn, which dilates blood vessels, is an ACE inhibitor (similar to prescriptions for high blood pressure like Lisinopril or Enalapril) and anti-oxidant and protects against artery damage by inhibiting plaque buildup on the arteries, and increases energy supply to the heart. Hawthorne Berries are a good preventative, as regular use has been shown to strengthen the heart muscle.

---

[75] Garlic can cause you to burp a garlic taste or smell like you've eaten a lot of it. I have used processed capsules of garlic like Kyolic for years. It is scentless and keeps you from smelling like you've had scampi 15 days in a row. You can open up the Kyolic capsules and mix the appropriate amount with your blend.

Ginkgo Biloba is a vasodilator, a circulatory stimulant and anti-inflammatory. Ginkgo improves circulation, has a normalizing action on the circulatory system and relaxes blood vessels.

Valerian Root is a sedative, which is good for relieving nervousness and tension, and suppressing and regulating the autonomic nervous system. Stress is believed to be a big contributing factor to hypertension, so relaxation is very important in controlling the disease.

Peppermint Leaf has nothing to do with high blood pressure but can help calm the stomach from potential upset caused by the other herbs. Garlic can sometimes cause stomach upset and peppermint leaf, as a carminative and digestive aid, can help counteract that effect. Consider this an optional addition based upon your tastes.

Dosage and Administration[76]

I recommend using powdered forms of the herbs; they blend better that way and you can be sure you are getting the appropriate amount and combination of all the herbs in the formula. If you cannot purchase the herbs already powdered you can do it yourself in an electric coffee grinder.

You have two choices in making capsules: you can just scoop the herbs out of bowl with half the capsule and then close it up or you can get a capsule making device. I have a capsule maker that fills 50 capsules at a time. You can find these on line or in most health food stores. Empty gel

---

[76] Please note, I am not a medical doctor and do not diagnose or prescribe. The recommended herbal dosages were gathered from numerous professional herbal books. Please consult a professional before ingesting herbs. Also if you are on prescription blood pressure medication, please consult your physician before trying these formulas as lowering your blood pressure too much has risks as well.

caps can also be obtained online, in health food stores, or wherever you purchase bulk herbs. For example, www.herbalremedies.com sells both vegetarian and gelatin (animal material) capsules for around $7 a pack.

After you have made your capsules, store them in a cool, dry place and keep them away from pets and children. I suggest taking two capsules, three times a day with meals which seems to be the average that my sources have recommended. Also consider altering your diet and increasing exercise to help lower your blood pressure.

Environmental Pollution
(A case study with a solution)

Martin was born and raised in Pittsburgh in the 1950's. It was a steel town and the air quality was horrible. Martin suffered from sinus problems and asthma but at that time no one was really concerned with the effects of pollution. He drank water from the tap that had high levels of lead and fluoride and his mother made a lot of pre-packaged meals from boxes and mixes. As an adult living in Los Angeles, Martin still suffers from sinus, ear and asthma problems. He has experienced some strange illnesses involving hair loss, constipation and foul smelling breath. He had hair analysis done and was stunned to learn he had high levels of mercury, aluminum and arsenic in his system. It was at this point he came to see me.

When most people think of environmental pollution they think of things they can see, like smoke from industrial plants, and exhaust from cars. What we are realizing today is that environmental pollution is everything from chemicals in our air and water, preservatives and dyes in our food to the additives in our shampoos, cosmetics and deodorants. Our soils are depleted and vegetables are covered in pesticides. Our cows and chickens are injected with hormones and antibiotics; we are bombarded with pollution that we never even considered was there.

Pollution can cause a litany of problems, from cancer to headaches to autoimmune diseases. It can make us tired and depressed or hyper and distracted. It affects every system of our body and can put a huge strain on our liver which is our main detoxifying organ. Part of the digestive system, the liver manufactures bile, digests worn out blood cells and bacteria, and stores fat. The liver is the largest gland in the body and is the only internal organ capable of regenerating itself.

It is virtually impossible for us to live on this planet today and not have some level of toxic exposure. The water, the air, the food, and just about every aspect of our lives has some sort of chemical component. Even the things in our homes such as carpets, plastics, and paint have an out gassing of chemicals that can remain in our bodies and negatively affect our health. I am not suggesting moving to the Amazon, living in a hut and growing and killing our own food, but being smart about what we put in and around our bodies.

So you see it is not only important to be a healthy consumer, but to use natural detoxification products for our bodies. No matter how healthy you try to be, everyone can benefit from an occasional detox. Herbal supplements and cleanses can also be extraordinarily beneficial to our health. A detox gives our cells a chance to release toxins and our liver a break to regenerate. It can eliminate disease and help us to recover more quickly in the future.

Cousins[77] (pg. 182) states "...research shows that when the intestinal toxemia is removed, symptoms such as fatigue, nervousness, gastrointestinal conditions, impaired nutrition, skin manifestations, endocrine disturbances, headaches, sciatica, various forms of low back pain, allergy, eye, ear, nose and throat congestion, even cardiac abnormalities have been healed in hundreds of cases."

But back to my client Martin. I suggested that he start taking some detoxifying herbs. I sent him to a doctor that does chelation therapy to help eliminate the metals in his system and told him that I would design an herbal formula for general cleansing.

Martin was a tea drinker so I decided to make a tea (decoction) containing equal amounts of the following herbs:

---

[77] Cousins, Gabriel, M.D. (2000) Conscious Eating, Berkeley, CA: North Atlantic Books.

Dandelion Root, Milk Thistle, Yellow Dock, Burdock Root, Fenugreek, Ginger, Parsley and Fennel. [78] [79] [80] [81] [82]

<u>Dandelion Root</u> is a powerful diuretic which is beneficial to the liver and eliminates toxins from the blood. It is also useful for clearing obstructions from the spleen, pancreas, gall bladder, bladder and kidneys.

<u>Milk Thistle</u> is used to support the liver, gall bladder and spleen. It protects the liver if taken before food and alcohol consumption.

<u>Yellow Dock</u> tones the entire system and improves the flow of bile.

<u>Burdock Root</u> is used to neutralize and expel toxins from the body and improves kidney function.

<u>Fenugreek</u> is used for lung support and combined with Milk Thistle, supports liver function.

<u>Ginger</u> has a cleansing effect on the bowels, skin and kidneys. It also adds a pleasant taste to the tea.

<u>Parsley</u> is a diuretic and cleans the liver of toxic waste.

---

[78] Daily Detox Tea. Retrieved April 7, 2007 from website: www.wholeapproach.com

[79] Liver Detox Tea. Retrieved April 7, 2007 from website: www.care2.com

[80] Liver Detox Tea. Retrieved April 7, 2007 from website: www.herbalfitness.com/liver

[81] Liver Detox Tea. Retrieved April 7, 2007 from website: www.localharvest.org

[82] Tenney, Louise M.H. (1992) Today's Herbal Health (Third Edition), Provo, UT: Woodland Books.

<u>Fennel</u> helps remove waste from the body and is also pleasant tasting.

I combined all the herbs which I purchased in the cut form since powder can get messy when making teas. I mixed the herbs well and made them into tea bags. (I found a health food store that sells empty tea bags that can be stuffed and then sealed using an iron.) I suggested 3 cups of tea per day steeped for 15 minutes, for 1 month.

Between the detoxifying herbal blend, the chelation therapy and slight diet changes, Martin felt better. Not only did his asthma disappear but his sinus difficulties diminished.

A Whole Body Herbal Tonic

In our Western medical lingo, we don't regularly hear the word tonic. When we do we either think of snake oil and traveling salesmen or a mixer for our gin. But taking medicinal tonics has been popular for thousands of years. They are meant to be taken regularly and strengthen the immune system, restore energy, aid digestion, nourish the blood and counteract the negative effects of living on this planet.[83]

Below is a list of beneficial herbs that all make wonderful tonics. I recommend using equal parts of all to make a well rounded tonic for overall health. I chose these herbs from numerous sources, not only because of their tonic properties but also for the nutritive and organ supporting power. The specifics on each herb follow.

Alfalfa contains health building properties, is high in vitamins and trace minerals, eliminates retained water and contains chlorophyll and enzymes that neutralize cancer in the system. It is a great source of protein and fights infection.

Dandelion is a powerful diuretic and blood purifier that supports the kidneys and liver. It is also a good source of vitamins and minerals.

Ginger is a very effective cleansing agent through the bowels, kidneys and skin. It enhances the effectiveness of other herbs, is good for the respiratory system, digestion and headaches, aches and pains and is high in protein, vitamins and minerals. Ginger is inexpensive, effective and widely available.

---

[83] http://www.ecosalon.com/the_history_of_tonics/

Gotu Kola is a traditional blood purifier, tonic and diuretic. It increases mental and physical power, combats stress, improves brain function, helps the body defend against various toxins and can help prevent against nervous breakdown.

Kelp is another important herb not just for its tonic power but for its ability to fight numerous diseases. Kelp has been shown to lower breast cancer rate, improve blood pressure, thyroid deficiency, constipation, gastrointestinal problems and infectious disease. Kelp also contains nearly 30 minerals and is a good supporter of glandular health.

Siberian Ginseng has been used in Chinese medicine for over 2000 years. Its benefits are numerous including being an anti-cancer agent, improving vision and hearing, and reducing depression and stress. It also has the adaptogenic ability to raise blood pressure and glucose levels when low and lower them when high.

Suma, known as Para Todo (for all things), is known to heal and prevent disease. [84] Suma is also an adaptogen and can inhibit tumor cell growth, promote healing of wounds and new cell growth, regulate blood sugar levels, stimulate the immune system, and has analgesic and anti-inflammatory properties. It is very valuable nutritionally, containing high amounts of vitamins, trace minerals and 19 amino acids.

I recommend buying whole or cut herbs as freshly dried as possible, powdering them and taking them in capsule form. Powdered herbs lose their potency quickly so buying pre-powdered herbs isn't always as effective. I suggest two capsules, three times per day with meals. More can be taken if feeling run down or recovering from illness. Do not take if pregnant or breastfeeding. And as with all

---

[84] Retrieved April 21, 2007 from website
www.herbmed.com/sumaroot.html

natural remedies, consult your doctor before beginning any health program.

Book References

Balch, Phyllis CNC (2002) *Prescription for Herbal Healing*, NY: Avery Books.

Green, James (2000) *The Herbal Medicine-Makers Handbook*, CA: Crossing Press.

Mowrey, Daniel Ph.D (1986) *The Scientific Validation of Herbal Medicine*, New Canaan, CT: Cormorant Books.

Tenney, Louise M.H. (1992) *Today's Herbal Health* (Third Edition), Provo, UT: Woodland Books.

How to Stay Sick List –
The Keys to Non-Healthy Living

I believe that our stories become our bodies and what we say to and about ourselves, becomes ourselves. So…if you want to stay sick, here's how.

Tell everyone you meet how horrible your life is. Make it an identity instead of an anecdote.

Find other negative people and make them your best friends.

Blame luck for everything, then you have no personal responsibility.

Say "why me?" a lot.

Live in the past, think a lot about the bad stuff and tell everyone.

Fear the future. You know it's going to suck!

Take no risks to grow and evolve.

Ask for things that will help you and then ignore them or do them half way.

Don't relax; after all, you're very busy.

Make excuses like: after the kids leave home, when I'm older, I'm too young…

Believe that what you think has no effect on the body.

Believe your illness/sickness is hereditary and you have no control.

Remember there are never EVER options for the future.

Stay in a job you don't like, or with a spouse you can't stand.

Never laugh, it's for idiots.

Resent people from your past and blame them for who you are now.

Put yourself down at every turn. You truly are all those things you say.

Tell everyone how useless you are and use words like "never" & "always".

Blindly take every prescription that your doctor gives you assuming he has your best interest at heart.

Surround yourself with negativity by watching the news and reading the paper often.

Don't stretch, eat right, breathe, drink enough water, poop, exercise or get any body work done.

Eat too fast when you are stressed and upset and don't chew.

Ask to be cured and not healed.

Envy everyone else for what you don't have.

Consume a lot of chemicals in food, water, air and home products.

Focus on all your problems.

Try to live up to what others think you should be, ignoring your own goals and desires.

Apologize for existing.

Let fear guide you and keep you stuck.

Hold on to your anger and negative emotions.

Try to fix everyone else, they're broken.

***Remember, you can never change!

How to Stay Healthy List
A Better Choice

Tell people of your successes and accomplishments. They can learn from you.

Find positive, supportive people and leave the negative behind you.

Take personal responsibility.

Know that others have bad times too, you're not alone.

Live in the present moment. Don't dwell on the past or fatalize about the future.

Go forward into the future with a positive attitude. It's going to be phenomenal.

Take risks to grow and evolve.

When you are gifted with something you asked for. Be thankful and follow through.

Relax.

Don't make excuses. The time is now.

Know that what you think has profound influence on your body.

You don't have to be your heredity. Perhaps there is another choice.

There are always options for the future.

Find a way to remove yourself from bad situations like jobs or partners. Or at least, change your attitude.

Laugh.

Don't blame or resent people from your past. Healing comes from forgiveness and moving forward.

Speak only positively about yourself.

Don't use words like "never" and "always".

Check into your prescriptions before you take them. Do your own research.

Take a news fast and let the paper and newscasts go for a few days.

Stretch, eat right, drink enough water, have healthy bowels and have body work done.

Eat slowly, in a calm environment and chew your food thoroughly.

Find true healing; don't just rely on a cure.

Healing: Physiology or Attitude?

I wrote this after I suffered a back injury as a means of exploring my thoughts, beliefs, attitudes and questions about healing. I have included this free form monologue, as I believe it offers some insight into natural healing.

How is it that people are diagnosed with the same dis-orders or dis-eases and some recover quickly while others spend years wallowing in their problems? Do we develop the cold because we feel a sniffle and say to ourselves "Oh great, we're getting a cold?" How is it that I can injure a disk and in telling myself "I'll be fine in a week", be fine. Others struggle for years with disc problems, with seemingly no light at the end of the tunnel. How is it that of 100 asymptomatic patients through MRI are shown to have herniated or bulging discs and be pain free and other suffer ad infinitum? I want to explore these issues and discover how the mind affects the healing process.

I healed a cracked vertebra when I was in college, I also believed I could. I started scheduling my clients a week after my arthroscopic knee surgery. I was ready to go in that week, where I heard of others that spent weeks in bed after the exact same surgery. Is it the doctor, the body type, the resilience of the patient? How much does attitude play a part in healing? What is "eating at" the person with the ulcers? What is "getting under the skin" of the person with psoriasis? How many hearts are breaking? How many people have their "hands full" and end up with carpal tunnel? Have the weight of the world on their shoulders and have chronic back and neck pain? What can be done about this?

It certainly isn't about Western medicine's pharmacopeia of solutions. How many more drugs must we take to offset the side effects of the first pill? Can we not convince our bodies to heal ourselves? If some can . . . why can't everyone? Do people truly want to be well? What would they talk about at parties if they were healthy and happy? How would they get the attention they desire if it wasn't for the pain that kept them locked up and brought down? Can we be truly healthy without taking responsibility for our own healing?

Does it make a difference that after my back injury I went right back to work? I cancelled no clients; I didn't lie in bed or run to the Western medicine cabinet. Did I have moments of fear? I certainly did and then my husband reminded me that I'm not those people in chronic pain. I am strong and can over come. I went to the chiropractor. I stretched....oh so much... I had massage, I used crystals and reiki and positive self talk and less than a week later, I was left with a bit of muscle tension and nothing else. Was it my mind, my perseverance, the not giving in to the pain...or did I just not hurt myself very much? Who determines how much we hurt? If people are walking around with all these horrible structural maladies and never feel any pain or symptoms, what makes them different than those non-functioning people with lesser disorders?

People seem to not want to take responsibility for their own actions, their mistakes, their healing. They walk into the doctor's office and want the magic pill to take all their worries away. They opt for surgery rather than a stretching and exercise routine. The easy way out...Then when it doesn't work, because they go back to the same unhappiness or same bad posture, they blame the doctor. Fix me. Well, have you stretched...no. Have you been exercising ...no. Have you been drinking water, watching your posture, cutting out dairy, taking your supplements, not smoking, not doing drugs, not sitting on your wallet, not beating your kids.......NO....fix me!

The reality is people just have to fix themselves. And it's not easy and it takes work. And it's ultimately the only choice for healing.

Today's Brilliance

This was written for a contest. I was not selected but wanted to include this because I think the ideas presented are valuable. We were asked to write what brilliance we wanted to leave our fellow man.

If I could impart one important lesson to others, it would be that each and every one of us has choices in how we live our daily lives, and we create our own reality with thoughts and actions.

It would be completely unacceptable for someone to follow us around insulting us every two minutes, telling us we're not good enough, we're fat, we're ugly, we're stupid, or that we are going to fail. But this is often exactly what we say to ourselves.

Yes, change is scary and with true health comes great personal responsibility. It is much easier to stay sick. When we are sick, very little is expected of us. We get pity and we get privileges. When we are healthy, we are expected to be present, show up at work, help others and to not play the constant role of victim that is so common in our society.

I want to encourage, to educate and to enlighten. I want to tell people about self-love and the power they all have within themselves. I want people to let the fear go, to embrace the inner authority that exists in each of us in order to make better, stronger, healthier choices. Choose to be around others who encourage growth and choose to thrive in your own life and in your community.

The ability to transform this world starts with the individual; especially individuals who are changing, growing, evolving and loving. Take control and take back your power. If you don't live your life, then someone else will come in and live it for you: the government, your doctor, your spouse, your boss, the church. Ultimately, only you can govern you.

I have helped people heal on an individual level. I have spoken before groups and taught in classrooms about healing. But I want to help on a global level. I want to help people embrace the inner healer, that light within us all that shines into our body, mind and spirit. We no longer need the pain, we no longer need the misery, and we no longer need the debt. We are whole and can make beneficial changes that allow growth and evolution.

Carolyn Myss coined the phrase "woundology", which is a term depicting how we use our wounds as a method to speak and connect with people and seek their approval. The pattern of woundology is so prevalent that it can take effort to realize we can also relate through our strengths and that we no longer need to hide behind our lack. Suffering is not growth and change does not come through complaining. Walking the path of healing is difficult, but we ALL have the ability to choose that path.

I want to be the roadmap to that path, to instill confidence in people of all ages that change is possible and through change comes growth, enlightenment and independence. We all have it! We all can do it! Let it shine through!

About the Author

Kathy Gruver has two decades of hands on experience and has earned her Doctorate as a Traditional Naturopath, her Masters in Natural Health and is pursuing her PhD. She graduated Cum Laude with a BFA in theatre from Point Park University in Pittsburgh and was a working actor in Los Angeles for many years. She serves on the faculty of SBBCollege where she teaches massage, nutrition and pathology. She has lectured for both the public and universities. Kathy has produced, directed and hosted an instructional massage DVD, *Therapeutic Massage at Home; Learn to Rub People the **RIGHT** Way!*

Kathy has worked with thousands of clients as young as 6 and as old as 103. She has helped people heal, not only on physical level, but emotionally and spiritually as well. Kathy has assisted with both births and end of life transitions.

Gruver has been featured as an expert is publications such as Massage Magazine, SouthWest Blend, Discover, First for Women, SB Fitness, The Holistic Option, Bottled Water Web, DermaScope Magazine, and Pacific Coast Business Times. She has written dozens of health and wellness articles and has appeared as a guest on over 30 radio shows covering topics such as back pain, mind/body medicine, healthy pregnancy, homeopathics, nutrition, herbs, patient advocacy and massage for wellness.

Kathy serves on the advisory committee for The Holistic Option, a website resource for all your natural health and wellness needs. She was their featured expert on a podcast on the Emotional Components of Back Pain. And her business Healing Circle Massage was featured as a Best Practice by Massage Magazine two years in a row.

Kathy lives in Santa Barbara with her husband and 2 cats.

Index

Recommended Reading and Resources

Bach Flower Therapy, Mechthild Scheffer, 1988.

Today's Herbal Health, Louise Tenney, MH, 2000.

Everybody's Guide to Homeopathic Medication, Cummings and Ullman, 1997.

You Can Heal Your Life, Louise Hay, 2004.

Memory Minder: A personal health journal, Memory Minder Journals, 2005.

Your Right to Know, Andrew Kimbrell, 2007. This is a great book about genetically modified foods and what corporate farming is doing to our food supply.

Hands of Light, Barbara Ann Brennan, 1987.

Essential Reiki, Diane Stein, 1996.

Stretching, Bob Anderson, 1980.

Myofascial Pain and Dysfunction, The Trigger Point Manual, Travell and Simons, Lippincott, Williams and Wilkins, Philadelphia, 1984.

Healing Back pain, John Sarno, 1991.

Mind over Back Pain, John Sarno, 1982.

A-Z Guide to Drug-Herb-Vitamin Interactions, Edited by Alan Gaby and Healthnotes Medical Team, 2006.

Prescription for Herbal Healing, Phyllis Balch, 2002.

Prescription for Nutritional Healing, Phyllis Balch, 1997.

Heal your Body A-Z, Louise Hay, 1998.

Dr. Jensen's Guide to Better Bowel Care, Dr. Bernard Jensen, 1999.

The Wellness Book, Benson and Stuart, 1993.

8 Weeks to Optimum Health, Andrew Weil, 1997.

150 Healthiest Foods on Earth, Jonny Bowden, 2007.

The Spirit of Homeopathic Medicines, Didier Grandgeorge, 1998.

DVDs

The Future of Food, Deborah Koons Garcia, 2004.

Prescription for Disaster, Gary Null, 2005.

You Can Heal Your Life, Louise Hay, 2007.

Super Size Me, Morgan Spurlock, 2004.

Food, Inc., Robert Kenner and Eric Schlosser, 2009.

Sweet Misery: A Poisoned World, Cori Brackett, 2004.

The Business of Being Born, Ricki Lake, Abby Epstein, 2007.

The Beautiful Truth, Cinema Libre Studios and Steve Kroschel, 2008.

Therapeutic Massage at Home; Learn to Rub People the RIGHT Way!, Kathy Gruver, 2009.

Pellinore
1992-2010

As I finished writing this book and was about to
send it to print, my cat Pellinore had to be put to
sleep after a battle with renal failure. Since he sat
in my lap through my writing this entire book,
I had to pay tribute to him here.

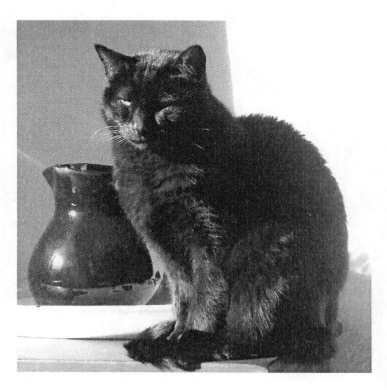

P-man, we will miss you!